Dedication

For all of us on a healing journey. Especially dedicated to all the people who we have had the privilege of teaching, and the honor of holding the sacred space for wisdom to reveal itself. You truly are our teachers.

To Sally
Thank you for being part of this book.
May the ripple effect of these stories
bring more healing to the world.

Guided Imagery
and Beyond

Stories of Healing and Transformation

Susan Ezra, RN, HN-BC and Terry Reed, RN, MS, HN-BC
Edited by Jan Maxwell, RN, BA, HN-BC

Susan Ezra & Terry Reed

Outskirts Press, Inc.
Denver, Colorado

Guided Imagery and Beyond
Stories of Healing and Transformation

Outskirts Press, Inc.
http://www.outskirtspress.com

ISBN: 978-1-4327-1974-6

Outskirts Press and the "OP" logo are trademarks belonging to Outskirts Press, Inc.

Disclaimer

The material presented in the stories contained in this book reflect the individual's ideas and choices and are the sole responsibility of the imagery guide and/or the client/patient.

The graduates of Beyond Ordinary Nursing have been trained to use Integrative Imagery within their scope of practice and to use it as an adjunct to standard medical care, not as a replacement. It is recommended that any intervention, including imagery, be provided by a trained and/or licensed healthcare professional.

Table of Contents

Acknowledgments   xi
Integrative Imagery Poem   xiii
Foreword   xv
Introduction   xvii
Prologue   ixx

Section One   In The Realm Of The Imagination   1
Section Two   Sacred Stories From Many Souls   15

Imagery For Personal Growth   17
    An Eagle Named Wind   18
    Peaceful Presence   23
    Wrapped In A Blanket Of Trust   25
    Freeing Trauma From The Past And Present   29
    A Very Special Place   31
    Blue Shoes   33

Imagery For Personal Development   39
    Transforming The Cage   40
    Being Erin Brochovich   43

Creating A New Job With Cautious John And Creative John   45
To Be Or Not To Be....Famous   49
Embracing The Fire   52

Imagery For Childbirth   57
   The Littlest Angel   58
   A Mom Ready For Her Twins   61

Imagery In Living And Dying   65
   With The Help Of The Choir   66
   Being Brave Enough To Offer   69
   Grief Can Be Bearable   71
   Our Lady Of Guadalupe Claims Her Own   74
   On The Other Side Of The Bridge   78

Imagery For Health And Wellness   83
   Healing From Within   84
   The Power Of Example   88
   Messages From Jesus   90
   Things Are Not Always What They Appear To Be   92
   A Moment In Time   95

Imagery For Cancer And Treatment   99
   The Owl And The Eagle   100
   Carolyn's Angel   105
   A New View Of Chemotherapy   108
   Wisdom For Making A Difficult Decision   110
   My Guides   113

Imagery For Pain Relief   117
   Little Green Inch Worm As Healer   118
   A True Experience Of Transforming Pain   120
   A Bough Heavy With Snow   123
   Better Than Drugs!   127
   Numbing The Pain Away   129
   Playing With Flipper   131

Imagery With Kids   133
   Mystic Knows The Song   134
   Sleeping In My Own Bed   137
   From Frightened To Fearless   139
   Blue Dragon Brings Relaxation And Freedom   142

Section Three The Ripple Effect   147
   A Dream Only An Image Away   150
   Transforming Images into Reality   154
   Accessing Financial Wisdom Through Imagery   156
   Confessions Of A Reluctant Therapist   159
   Blending Shamanic Healing With Imagery   162
   Stress Relief For Stressed-out Nurses   165
   An Idea Whose Time Has Come: Hospital-based Imagery   167

Section Four References and Resources   173
   References   175
   BON Certificate Program in Imagery   177
   Professional Associations   179
   Certified Imagery Practitioners   179
   Guided Imagery CDs   179
   Bibliography   181

Acknowledgments

It is said that gratitude is a spiritual practice.

We bow deeply with appreciation and gratitude to all the contributors to this book for sharing their stories from the heart. They include Julie Bernard, Patty Buch, Dottie Burdine, Ginger Carr, Joan Costello, Nancy Cox, Kathy Darlington, Sylvia Domagalski, Glenda Ericson, Jann Fredrickson, Miranda George, Donna Guyot, Cheryl Hann, Jennifer Hetherington, Denise Hughes, Esther Johnson, Mary Ellen Kinney, Sally Lippitt-Houston, Jan Maxwell, Deborah McElligott, Lynn McKeon, Pat Merritt, Sandra Roberts, Debbie Smith, Judy Sweet, Roxanne WhiteLight and Pat Wooldridge.

These stories are representative of hundreds of stories and imagery sessions. Therefore, we also wish to acknowledge every one of our students and graduates. And thanks to Nanci Warner for the Integrative Imagery poem.

Jan Maxwell deserves the greatest praise for without our "amiga" the stories would not have been so lovingly coaxed into being and edited with such refinement. She started this journey with us so many years ago and now has had a significant hand in bringing this book to fruition. We *really* could not have done this without Jan.

We honor our faculty: Linda, Donna, Ginny and Kathy, and all our fellow mentors/teachers who have shared in our vision and adventures, and have played an integral role in transforming the vision into a reality. Each individual has made an indelible imprint upon Beyond Ordinary Nursing with a unique contribution of knowledge, wisdom and wit. To all of you we are greatly indebted.

It is a blessing to have Linda Hershenson as our administrative assistant. She has made the administrative tasks easy to bear and share. Her eagle eye and mind for detail has helped immensely in the advancement of the book and the teaching program. Carol Kinney is recognized, as well, for assisting us for five years, especially with the Hawaii conference. And hail to Liz Rieden who believed in us from the very beginning.

Thank you to our predecessors, and pioneers such as Jeanne Achterberg, Barbara and Larry Dossey, Emmett Miller, Rachel Remen and Tak Poon, who have forged the way ahead of us. A special heartfelt thanks to Belleruth Naparstek, who has befriended us and always models the feminine principle so stunningly; she is our *hero*.

We express the deepest appreciation to our teachers David Bresler and Marty Rossman who started us on our amazing adventure into the realm of imagery. They are true visionaries and leaders in the advancement of imagery as a crucial component of CAM (Complementary and Alternative Medicine). Their foresight has forged a path for many to follow.

Integrative Imagery

Wisdom lies within/
Language/
for which there are no words,/
Only symbols./
Going within/
to the Source./
Connecting with inner wisdom./
The alignment of reality/
in the physical realm,/
with the spiritual laws/
of metaphysical wisdom./

Holding the space sacred/
for the journey./
Fully present./
Loving, not judging./
Allowing, not prescribing./
Opening the door/
to wonder,/
possibility/
and wholeness./

Nanci L.Warner
8/15/99
Tucson, AZ
Phase IV
Graduation

Foreword

This is a book whose time has surely come. Guided imagery, once considered a marginal practice on the outer fringes of alternative medicine, has made its way into mainstream medicine in the space of a mere decade or two. Research has established its efficacy and usefulness for stress, anxiety, pain, insomnia, neuromuscular rehabilitation, cardiac health, improved intellectual performance, posttraumatic stress and better tolerance of medical procedures, particularly surgery and chemotherapy. Now delivered as a commonplace intervention in hundreds of hospitals, health plans and employee assistance programs, it continues to impress providers as it reassures and empowers users.

Susan Ezra and Terry Reed, co-founders of Beyond Ordinary Nursing, are two of the reasons why, in such a short space of time, guided imagery has achieved such an accelerated legitimacy in the world of traditional healthcare. Taught and trained by Interactive Guided Imagery[sm] pioneers, Martin Rossman and David Bresler, at the legendary Academy for Guided Imagery, these two passionate enthusiasts have introduced imagery to scores of nurses and other health professionals, expanding the field and contributing to a more compassionate, personal, empowering delivery of health services, nationwide.

Luckily for the rest of us, in the course of their teaching, they have collected the wonderful, inspiring, personal stories you are about to read in this book. Not only do these accounts motivate better, wiser use of this magical, internal process; they also illuminate its elegant simplicity, creativity and range; and demonstrate how astonishingly easy it is to use. Without these stories, it would be hard to believe how powerful and even life-changing this simple, gentle technique is. Nothing drives the point home better than these heartfelt accounts.

And for those readers who hunger for the science behind the magic, they will find this here as well. Susan and Terry provide a satisfying overview of how and why imagery works. They also put it in historical perspective and compare and contrast its different but related techniques.

This is a book for both practitioners and health consumers, reminding all of us of the primacy of our imaginations and the power of turning inward. In this age of high tech healthcare, this high touch approach is badly needed.

Belleruth Naparstek, LISW
Psychotherapist and founder of Health Journeys
Author of Invisible Heroes: Survivors of trauma and how they heal

Introduction

*There are no days in life so memorable as those which vibrate
to some stroke of the imagination.*
                                                    ~Ralph Waldo Emerson

This book is about transformation. Imagery is the vehicle. Contained within these pages are dozens of life-changing stories from Beyond Ordinary Nursing (BON), a training program in Integrative Imagery for healthcare professionals. The stories are from the founders of BON, the amazing people who have gone through the program and the clients who have been touched by the power of this work. Many of the stories are in the client's own words.

After eleven years of teaching the Certificate Program in Imagery to hundreds of healthcare professionals, there comes a calling to compose some of the transformative stories in the shape of a book in order to share this work with even more people, both healthcare practitioners and the broader community. Just as with all aspects of the evolution of our program, this book has been guided by the hand of the divine. It is as if the stories are calling out to be heard by others. We all know that stories heal. Storytelling is as old as the human community. In fact, our souls crave stories that teach and guide and heal. It has been said that sometimes we need a story more than food.

The stories in this book tell of the transformative power of Integrative Imagery and in that way they educate. You, as the reader, might choose one story at a time or choose to read all of them. They illuminate the amazing wisdom and noetic, or intuitive, knowledge that resides within each one of us. As such, this book is not intended to be a self-help or how-to-book, nor is it formulated to be a scholarly or researched-based text for there are many books serving that purpose.

All of the contributions are from real people in real life situations-some dramatic, some mundane. Several are examples of documented sessions demonstrating the techniques required for certification. The reader may notice a difference in the style from the documented session stories and the stories written specifically for the book. The documented sessions follow a specific format and often include actual dialogue. They show the power of imagery and the magical things that can happen even with relatively new guides and clients who are using the imagery process for the first time. We have also included some brief, quick interventions. The stories are as close to the original as possible, with some revisions for cogency and conciseness. Confidentiality is maintained with pseudonyms in all of the stories, unless requested otherwise. We have attempted to give a sampling of many and diverse ways imagery can transform and heal. This book illustrates that we are all ordinary people with extraordinary abilities, if we choose to use them.

Mostly, we wish this book to inform and inspire the mind, heart and soul of each reader.

Prologue

The meaning of our existence is not invented by ourselves, but rather detected.

~Viktor Frankl

Manifesting Our Dream Into Reality
The Story of Beyond Ordinary Nursing (BON)

All stories have a beginning. It is important for us to tell our story of the inception and evolution of BON, because the company is an example of a successful business developed and administered by nurses. Nurses, like many women, are often limited by society's roles or job descriptions. Women, as well as men, need models of success and independence. BON also represents a partnership of extra-ordinary collaboration and friendship, a model that is unusual in this corporate, competitive environment in which we live, be we women or men. Additionally, BON reflects the growth and development of its two co-founders. It is significant to tell our personal story as well. One cannot really separate personal from professional, for one is mirrored in the other. As it is within, so it is without. What has been true for us is very likely relevant for others and we hope others can delight in and relate to our experience. Indeed, we all need stories to guide us and spur us on.

Florence Nightingale, the mother of nursing, spoke of a *"must"* that each one of us are called upon to do in our lifetime. Bringing imagery into healthcare has become our life's purpose, our *must*. We want to inspire others to believe that they, too, can listen to their calling, trust it and have the courage to act upon it. When we do this, the divine always hears and responds. Florence Nightingale is an archetype for this. Being born into a life of prestige and privilege, she followed her life-long determination to bring holistic health practices, spiritual principles and basic hygiene (which was minimally existent in the 1800's) into medical practice. In her 90-year life span she established nursing as a credible, viable, valuable profession. As Barbara Dossey, PhD, RN and Nightingale scholar, articulates, "Florence was a true scientist, visionary, mystic and healer." This is our legacy in nursing to which we can aspire. Each of us, in all fields of healthcare, is challenged to bring our passion into our practice. This alone could transform care everywhere. Moreover, all of us, not just in healthcare, are challenged to heed the calling to fulfill our life purpose. Along the road, it serves us all to hear the lessons learned from our fellow sojourners.

Our Inspiration

We have been talking about our *must;* that which gives meaning and purpose to life. Dreams can start very early, but until we pay attention to them, they may lay dormant for many years or even a lifetime. In our case, the dream was born in imagery and once conscious, could not be denied or postponed. The energy was persistent, pushing us forward with increasing urgency and fire. This glimpse and connection to our life's passion was critical, as the journey of bringing our dreams into reality would propel us far beyond our comfort zones.

For Susan and Terry, the ten-year journey that was celebrated in 2006 with an imagery conference, most likely started very early in life, but more recently the pivotal event that brought us together was our imagery training with the Academy for Guided Imagery

(AGI). We were both already holistic nurses, Susan working in hospice and private practice and Terry working in critical care and private practice. The imagery training felt like a "hand in glove" and gave both of us the formal structure to facilitate the healing work in which we so strongly believed.

We have been trained by and have taught with the Academy for Guided Imagery, which was the first of its kind to develop a core curriculum in this powerful, individualized form of guided imagery. The origins of this pioneering work can be traced to the theories of luminaries like Drs. Carl Jung, Irving Oyle and Roberto Assagioli. In 1989, the Academy was co-founded by David Bresler, PhD and Marty Rossman, MD who were the first to give name and structure to this system of using imagery. They termed it Interactive Guided Imagery[sm].

During our faculty training at AGI, we met another kindred soul, Jan Maxwell, also a holistic nurse in private practice who had been trained to use imagery. So it was no surprise that we began to share our dreams of teaching nurses to bring imagery to their patients. We created a weekend training program that came effortlessly into form. We knew we were doing pioneering work together and knew imagery would be a profound tool that could change nursing from a fix-it model to a self-care model with healing rather than curing as the focus. We called ourselves the "tres amigas," a name we still use with each other. It was soon after the success and excitement of the weekend training that the idea of a full imagery certification program for nurses was born.

While Jan made a hard decision not to move forward with creating a very time-consuming certification program, she has continued to be our supporter, model of self-care, and now our editor.

Our Own History Lessons

It took us, Terry and Susan, a full year to move through a goal setting process that included becoming business partners. The answers to five questions we asked ourselves were vital in keeping us on track. We now share these questions and a process we call "Manifesting dreams into reality" used in the last phase of our imagery program.

Here are the questions and answers we used:

What do we want? (Our goal is) We will create a certificate program in imagery for registered nurses. We are self-employed and financially responsible for ourselves.

How long to get it? One year. Today is April 15, 1995. This will be completed on April 15, 1996.

Why do we want it? (What's in it for us?) We want to have the freedom to create a training program that "lives our philosophy." We want to have a greater impact on the world by teaching greater numbers of people. We want to feel free and not stifled by a bureaucratic system.

Why don't we have it now? (Obstacles or mind chatter) We don't think that it is possible to work for ourselves. We don't think that we can afford it. We are scared to give up the security of a stable job. Some people tell us that we cannot do it.

How can we get it? (Solutions) We can develop affirmations that build self-confidence. We can use imagery to keep us grounded and rehearse our vision. We can read books on creating a business. Once we are partners, we will form goals and plans. We can pray!

Our first workshop was on April 26, 1996, just eleven days past our target date!

Challenges

The hard and often tedious work of moving the free flowing and creative energy of imagery into the energy of manifestation can be likened to moving from daydreaming on a spring day to thunder clouds rolling across your inner landscape. In retrospect, it was a time of flow of the yin and yang, of dark and light; from impasse and resistance to success and profound gifts.

We knew we were going to have to stretch and move into unknown and scary territory. After a year of planning and many imagery sessions, Terry left her day job of 24 years. Grief and fear of letting go ran their course throughout most of the year. It felt like stepping off a cliff and being excited at the same time.

Susan was propelled into her own "dark night of the soul." The depth of this soul time required not only claiming power professionally, but the dissolution of a 30 year marriage. The challenge was not to stand in anyone else's shadow. Through her journey, she found that in the shadow lay her hidden power, the light as well as the dark.

In 1999, we made the decision to individuate as a company and end our contract with the AGI. While we were grateful for the support and help the Academy gave us in making our dream come true, it was time to stand on our own. We had several spiritual taps on the shoulder, which we could no longer ignore, telling us the time had come to move on. A monumental learning curve confronted us. We re-wrote the curriculum and took the necessary steps to be an independent training program.

Enter Terry's imaginary wisdom figure, Pierre, a macaw who represents wisdom, lightness and humor. On February 22, 1999, Susan and Terry were driving back from a workshop in Santa Barbara, CA. We decided to stop and take a contemplative walk on Pismo Beach. We were feeling the full responsibility of the decision to take our program in a new direction. Our feelings were not so much the fear and resistance that were present in the development of the program, but grieving and letting go of one form and moving into another.

True to our foundations with BON, we decided to invite the imaginary Pierre to come and help us with the "what now" questions. He usually comes into Terry's imagination upside down, flying backwards and communicates advice by acting out messages with humor. During boring meetings, he has done such things as walk on people's papers or mussing their hair and Terry even gets messages like "this too shall pass." This particular time he walked up behind us (Terry is sharing with Susan what is happening as we walk along the beach) and put his wings around us. We could feel his incredible warmth, his breathing and heartbeat against our back and an incredible sense of protection. He communicated that we were not alone and that we were walking our talk and that we were on the right path. We both felt the healing we needed to grow and expand along with the feeling of an ending and a new beginning. *It was at this point that we came upon about 100 sand dollars on the beach, whole and intact.* Terry always looked for unbroken sand dollars as a good omen. We did take a few to remind us of the profound healing imagery we had just experienced. This inner wisdom imagery was pivotal to a new creativity and new voice that has regrounded us many times as the journey has moved forward.

Were it not for our deep commitment and passion to bring this work into the world, the guidance of Spirit, the support of our teachers, students and each other, we would not have persevered.

Harvesting the Wisdom

We enter this present phase of our continued journey with clarity and the sense of having shed an old skin. What we learned might come around in another form, but at this point we are making conscious choices that integrate the wisdom from the past with the new. There is more openness to options and possibilities that may come from unknown sources. As the Inuit people say "There are two plans for every day: my plan and the Mysterys' plans."

It was important to claim and acknowledge what we had learned. For Susan, her archetype for this harvesting time was the wise woman. Some of the attributes are finding the gifts and gratitude even in the midst of the difficult. Her biggest life lesson was to "intention" what she wanted/needed and then to let go of the form and time frame in which it would come.

For Terry, the major learning was about trust and letting go of old beliefs. That took the form of realizing you never lose what you already have, looking at experiences with fresh eyes, and using her inner wisdom to mediate the chatter of her inner critic. In addition, she learned from her business partnership with Susan that she didn't have to do it all; to listen more and that Terry's way wasn't always the only way.

We have tried very hard to practice one tenet; to really walk our talk, and in that to be living examples of what we are learning. We support each other in keeping this in our daily work. We now are acquiring a deeper understanding of the universal law of abundance and the law of attraction. Our greatest rewards and lessons have come from the exceptional people we have met through our training program. We see what others are doing with the powerful tool of imagery and the infinite ways creativity is expressed. This, more than anything, keeps us on our path and informs our teaching.

Dr. Jean Watson, a visionary and holistic nurse theorist, succinctly expresses our vision of generativity in her quote, "Living the four fold way is to hear the inner call as to how to translate one's own unique talents and gifts into compassionate service. To lead via the four fold path is to paradoxically manifest one's full self while simultaneously transcending ego self; to open to connections, visions of the whole, that are greater than any one person but unite us all." [1]

Stewardship

BON is continuing to evolve. We have taken our accumulated personal and professional experience and look forward to the future with curiosity, even when it is unknown. We are continually working on moving away from scarcity to abundance, manifesting prosperity and solvency. More possibilities are on the horizon for BON faculty, mentors and graduates. The tenth year celebration at our 2006 Hawaii conference was a culmination and this book is the next level of expression of our work. The form in which it is evolving is not yet clear, however we know that for any living thing to remain vibrant, it must change and evolve. At this level, we are far more trusting of the mystery and know the invisible will emerge when the time is right. We trust that BON has and will continue to inspire and to give healing and sustainability to ourselves, our students and the world.

Section One:
In The Realm
Of The Imagination

Imagination is the living power and prime agent of all human per-
ception.

~ *Samuel Taylor Coleridge*

A wakening the power of the imagination within us may be the most important discovery any of us ever make. Within each of us lies a wealth of wisdom and reservoir of resources, waiting to assist us as individuals and as a collective. Imagery is alive and well inside all of us. If that were not true, we would have no Peter Pan or Harry Potter or Yoda! The world of the imagination is home for the beginnings of all forms of creativity, ideas, inventions, arts and discovery. Its very nature is healing to both spirit and soul. This book primarily focuses on the use of imagery for health and healing.

All ancient cultures are rooted in a strong belief in the imagination, mystery or the unknown. The imaginal realm is where the seeds of healing, on all levels, reside. Since primal times, human beings have ventured into this inner landscape to seek information, messages and resources to help those who are sick of body, emotions or spirit. The shaman or medicine person acts on behalf of the one in need, journeying into the realm of the imagination. All ancient and modern indigenous cultures actively used/use some form of imagery in their construct of health/illness. So in a very real sense, imagery has to be part of healing. There is not a culture, past or present, which does not have some form of imagery tied to spiritual beliefs.

Early Grecian culture embraced the significance of images, and believed them to be "real" not just in the mind but as real entities. Indeed, images "live" in the imagination, awaiting us to discover them. Our ancient ancestors grasped the inner and outer world of reality and knew how to bridge the worlds in healing rituals and dream temples. "The Greeks said the senses take in the world, subtract matter, and form an image in the psyche, which was their term for the Soul and which they believed lived in the heart." [2]

The subconscious speaks to us in symbols and metaphors that our bodies instinctively know how to convert into physical building blocks of healing. Imagery is a natural part of our thought process; it is simply how the right brain "thinks." While the other half of the brain conceptualizes in linear, logical thoughts, the right brain grasps and processes information in pictures, images, senses and feelings. The information from this source is noetic knowledge that is from a deeper, intuitive place than our intellectual knowledge. Imagery is the universal language of the mind/body/spirit/soul. It can provide us with insights and information from our deeper self, and connect us with divine guidance.

Imagery is, in fact, akin to the magical; "magic" meaning that which is mystical and metaphysical, that which is greater than us. Imagery comes from the root word "mage." A mage is a magician who practices magery. Place an "I" in front of the word and you have the magic of *imagery*. Many things are possible when we can tap into this realm of possibilities. To fantasize is to make the invisible *visible*. This is not just pretend or make-believe. Images hold meaning and energy within the human psyche. An image is real; real in the imagination, yet translatable into the real world. The power of this process lies in the image itself because the image contains the energy, the essence of what it represents. An example will serve to illustrate this point. A young woman's image of her creative force is a fountain flowing up from the earth, reaching high into the sky, overflowing, and bursting forth. Focusing on this image every day allows this young woman to harness the energy of this symbol to translate it into the creative force needed to become a successful artist.

An eloquent quote by Carl Jung, MD speaks to this. "The psychological mechanism for transforming energy is the symbol." Image in this context is equated with the word symbol, whether it is an external object or internal image. Religious icons contain power for a religious community. A spiritual symbol can have a profound effect on a believer. This was the case of a woman about to have surgery, as told by a nurse who took care of her. She wore a red cord around her waist, which she never removed. She believed she would die if this cord came off. Despite this information, the cord was inadvertently removed while she was in the surgical suite. The patient did not survive the operation, even though all seemed well and there were no apparent complications.

One could theorize that the reason the modern world is in such disarray is because the imaginal roots of the culture have been severed. A major shift occurred in the Middle Ages when magical thinking became identified with superstition and evil, and rational thought process was not only valued but reigned supreme. The imagination was not respected, rather it was feared and banished into the dark recesses of the mind. The 1500's brought the dawning of the Scientific Revolution, lead by Renee Descartes, and others, who believed in the mechanistic view of the body as a machine. A division was formed. This resulted in the well known "Cartesian split" in which reason was separated from creativity and mind divorced from body. This dominated scientific and medical thinking for nearly five hundred years. During the fourteenth century, the human faculty of the imagination was not empowered by sufficient rationality. Today the reverse is true. Now rationality is not empowered sufficiently by the imagination. [3]

Thankfully, in the twentieth and twenty-first centuries we are now seeing a reunion of medicine and magic. With incredible scientific advances, we are also experiencing the re-emergence of many time-honored healing modalities from many cultures and traditions. Imagery is one of them. It is a marriage of the best of both worlds.

Sources and Types of Therapeutic Imagery

Most forms of meditation, hypnosis and dream analysis use some kind of imagery process. The process may be active, in directly engaging with the images, or may be receptive in just letting images arise spontaneously. Tibetan meditations, for example, often focus on an image of a deity, contemplating certain qualities or powers. In actuality, just about any insight process uses some form of imagery. We have included some definitions that might be helpful to the reader:

Imagery: Imagery is a natural thought process, using one or more of the five senses and usually associated with emotions. Just as we all dream, we all use imagery to picture a scene in our mind's eye, remember a pleasant childhood memory or recall a favorite piece of music. The creative process in writing, painting or developing a new idea cannot take place without imagery. One first imagines, then one creates. For many years, athletes have been using imagery rehearsal to visualize the activity and the end outcome of their sport with recognizable advantages.

Guided Imagery: Guided imagery is a therapeutic process that facilitates working with the power of the imagination to positively affect mental attitude and potentiate positive outcomes. In general, this process is scripted, structured and directed by a practitioner. For instance, a group may be guided on a journey in a hot air balloon to view the landscape below and see the "big picture." Commercial audiotapes and CDs are also examples of scripted "guided" imagery. Most people in the general population and in health care are already familiar with this style. As a matter of fact, guided imagery is one of the most accepted complementary therapies in medical centers and hospitals worldwide.

Integrative Imagery: This model takes the therapeutic process to an even deeper level by eliciting and working with a person's own images, both positive and negative. This process is best facilitated by a practitioner, guiding a person to bring to mind an image for something, then directly engaging with this image, often in dialogue. For example, an image of healing is elicited. Then by communicating with this image, one may uncover what is needed in order to heal. This process is somewhat like conscious dreaming in that we are able to communicate and interact with symbolic representations of our inner self and glean information. Judie Heinschel, PhD, RN, describes this as a "lived experience" in that "it is an experience that occurs as the client interacts with images." [4]

Communication between the client and the inner images may be in an interactive dialogue or in a sense of "knowing," a more intuitive sensing. Each person's imagery process is unique to them. However, most people access "images" through one or more of the senses. The majority of the population is visual and will see, picture, or envision an image. Some have very elaborate scenes and figures. Kinesthetic imagers, on the other hand, will primarily feel or sense something without "seeing" anything at all. Musicians and singers will often have a strong auditory presence. Closing your eyes and concentrating on a favorite piece of music is one way to experience imagery. Overall, images can be seen, felt, heard, touched, smelled or sometimes even tasted. The more senses that are recruited the richer the experience.

The dialogue component is one of the most important factors that distinguishes Integrative Imagery from guided imagery. Direct interaction between the client and the images is dynamic and powerful, leading to insights and wisdom from within that is less common in a receptive "guided imagery" process. The dialogue between the client and the guide is also crucial. Generally, the "right" brain conceptualizes in images and the "left" brain formulates language. While experiencing the imagery process in the right brain and describing that experience verbally to the guide using left brain function, the client seems to have an integration of the experience at a much deeper level. The interactivity between the client and the images can happen by engaging in the imagery process without a guide and some do this very well. However, for most of us, an essential element in the depth and power of the work lies in the guide facilitating the process, bearing witness and holding a safe and sacred space for the client.

Interactive Imagery[sm] **or Interactive Guided Imagery**[sm]**:** In concept and structure, this imagery modality was developed by David Bresler, PhD and Marty Rossman, MD, co-founders of the Academy for Guided Imagery. It is very similar and is the predecessor of Integrative Imagery.

This specialty of the active and interactive process is primarily based on the body of works of Carl Jung, MD, (Active Imagination) Roberto Assagioli, MD (an Italian psychiatrist who developed Psychosynthesis) and Irving Oyle, MD (a Bolinas, CA based physician.)

Both Interactive and Integrative Imagery:
- Are client-centered, focused and directed, leading to client empowerment.
- Are non-scripted (or minimally scripted), using language with few words.
- Facilitate the client in accessing and interacting with his/her own images, resources and wisdom.

- Use dialogue/communication between client and images and client and guide.
- Fosters a sacred, safe and therapeutic space for the client to work.

In one of the few research studies of this interactive process, Judie Heinschel, PhD, RN, reported the outcome of ten client experiences. Five patterns of response emerged: major personal transformation, specific life changes, expanded awareness, healing, and the wholeness of the experience. One client stated "Unequivocally, it has to do with healing. You cannot separate a connection, an alignment, intercommunication with the self, from healing." [5]

Similar Models Using Imagery

Hypnosis: Hypnosis has many similarities to the imagery process. It is defined as a state of physical relaxation and heightened mental concentration, where the mind is focused internally and is open to suggestion. There are many schools of hypnosis. Some are very similar in the client-centered approach and non-directive style, while others are quite directive. Often people want to know if they will be in control if they are hypnotized.

Meditation: This is also a focused state of mental concentration, more passive than the other processes. The focal point in meditation may be the breath, a word, phrase, object, etc. The goal of meditation is not to clear the mind of all thoughts for that is a difficult, if not impossible goal. One simply allows thoughts to come and go. The aim is to reach a deeper level of awareness, neutrality and inner peace. Out of this emerges wisdom and compassion for oneself and others.

Integrative Imagery Techniques

This section will describe some of the imagery techniques referred to in the stories within this book. This will give the reader some understanding and context and is not meant to be instruction for the individual techniques. Full instruction and training is provided in our certification program called the Certificate Program in Imagery, referenced in the Resource section.

There are many techniques that are used in the Integrative Imagery process. The technique is chosen based on the issue presented by the client and how it can best be addressed. All of the techniques rely on the premise that there is wisdom and insight within our deeper self that can help us address our own issues. The technique, **Working With An Image,** is perhaps the quintessential technique, for in imagery we are always working with some kind of image. In this process, the issue is identified, be it pain, a symptom, a problem, or a conflict. Then in a relaxed state, the client forms an image in their imagination that represents the issue. In a step-by-step process, the client explores the image, noting its shape, size, color, qualities, feelings and what it conveys. The image may even be given a voice and communicate what it wants, needs, or has to offer. Information gleaned can be very helpful to the client. For instance, based on the notion that pain is a message from the body, an image for one client's chronic back pain was "a gray, cold, hard vise in her back." By opening communication, the client was able to verbalize to the image that "there are not supposed to be vises in my back!" The image conveyed that it could offer the client strength since *it* was so strong. This was a completely different meaning for the pain than the client had previously believed, so she was able to feel stronger inside as the pain softened some. Remarkably, the pain went from a level of 9 down to a level of 1 (using the visual analog scale of 10 = worst and 0 = none) during the session. Over time the pain became manageable.

Accessing our inner wisdom is essential to our health and personal growth. We so often forget to utilize that inner knowing or sometimes even believe we have it. Two techniques, **Inner Wisdom** and **Inner Healer**, are exquisite in bringing us in touch with intuitive knowledge. There is a wise part of all of us who guides us every step of the way along our life's journey. Intuition is a part of intelligence. Most everyone can relate to a "gut sense" or "intuitive hit" or even hearing an inner voice. By giving a form (an image) to this wisdom we can more easily develop a relationship with this part of ourselves. In this way, it can better inform and guide us.

There is absolutely no end to how this form may take shape in one's unique imagination: a wise old man named Methiades; an eagle; a band of animal allies; water flowing through a stream; a very versatile spirit called Esmeralda; a rock; or special tree; or the color purple. Each symbol carries a gift or guidance. Having a "form" for this wisdom allows us to more easily communicate and interact with it. Some people have developed a deep and ongoing relationship that lasts years or even a lifetime.

Accessing Inner Strengths is another technique in which we can draw upon strengths and inner qualities that have helped us in the past. These strengths and qualities enable us to get through a challenging occurrence in the present. We can learn to call up courage or compassion or whatever quality is needed. Through imagery exploration, we can re-experience a past time when we felt the desired quality strongly, then bring that quality forward with us through an embodied feeling and practice using it where we need it in a current situation. This way we call upon our life experiences and our strengths that have served us through previous challenges. There is a vast reservoir of positive resources inside all of us.

Human beings are made up of a collection of parts, roles and identities, called in psychology "sub-personalities." All the parts of the self have individual functions, needs, feelings, and a unique voice. Some we know, some we like and identify with, others we deny or banish to a realm well below our conscious awareness. Two examples that are more commonly known are the "inner critic" or the "inner child." When we identify and work with these many aspects of ourselves, self-acceptance, conflict resolution and ultimately, wholeness occurs. In *Parts Work,* the client calls forth an image that represents the identified part and then, through dialogue, the client has an opportunity to get to know and understand that part better. In a more complex technique called *Polarity Work*, two images that are the polarized aspects of an inner conflict are called forth in the imagination so that each part is able to "speak its mind" and be heard by the other part. This is powerful and enlightening work.

Lastly, *Transforming Pain* is a technique using drawing and imagery of pain at three levels: "worst;" "least;" and "gone."

Drawing here is not about being an artist; its purpose is to express a representation of one's experience of pain, including feelings and sensations. Through imagery, the client is then able to "transform" the pain in their imagination, thereby altering the mind's perception of pain. This creates a template for the mind/body to actualize a pain-free state. This technique is easily adapted for use with stress, anxiety, emotional pain, and even other physical problems.

Mind-Body Research and Imagery

Psychoneuroimmunology (PNI) is the mind-body science that is the foundation for how and why imagery works. Since the 1970's, with the advancement of neuroscience, knowledge has emerged that verifies that the central nervous system, the endocrine system and the immune system are not separate systems but, in fact, are interlinked. PNI represents the scientific study of the interaction of the mind, the nervous system and the immune system. This current paradigm presents a new way of thinking about outdated anatomy and physiology theories that separate the mind and the body.

For those who are imagery practitioners and educators it is important to know the basics of PNI and the holistic approach it represents in order to introduce the concepts of imagery to clients and patients. It is also important for clients and patients to understand the basics of PNI so they know how the use of imagery allows them to have control over decreasing the risks of disease and improving well-being.

Imagery is something we do all the time. It is an innate ability that has many applications. From imaginary playmates as children to inner critics as adults, we are continually creating stories in our mind. Unfortunately, we use our imagination more often to conjure stressful thoughts about the past, or to fantasize about terrible events in the future. These thoughts are so automatic that we can go for long periods of time worrying away, unaware of how we are feeling or what is occurring in our bodies. The body's response is the same whether the event is actual or imagined. When an individual worries about losing a job, for example, the body releases potent chemicals such as adrenaline and cortisol, as if the individual already was unemployed. The body also responds when a person is thinking of a special someone or happy event. The body releases healing bio-chemicals such as endorphins, in response to the positive emotions of love and joy.

Emotions, associated with thoughts or images, start a cascade of bio-chemicals called peptides. These messenger molecules send information throughout the body. For instance, someone may experience being cut off on the freeway, think "what a jerk" and feel the emotion of fear and anger. Signals, by way of peptides such as adrenaline, lead to physiologic changes of the "fight or flight" response, increasing blood pressure and heart rate. Behavioral responses such as making angry gestures and yelling often follow. This process is referred to as the mind-body connection. Peptides are the messenger molecules that travel throughout the body and receptors are the docking stations on the surface of the cells. The receptors are often referred to as the "locks" and the peptides as the "keys." The entire surface of all cells have many different receptors on them. When the receptor binds with its own unique peptide a link is created, like a key in a lock, that causes the peptide to change its shape allowing the chemical (with its information) to enter the cell.

Our bodies truly have an "inner pharmacy" which is greatly influenced by the imagination. We can either push the adrenaline button or turn on the endorphin button, depending on perceptions, behaviors, thoughts and self-talk. Through recent research, we now know the body is listening and responding. PNI research has shown that chronically high levels of stress hormones such as adrenaline and cortisol interfere with immune system function. This results in decreased numbers of lymphocytes and killer T cells which defend the body against infection and disease. [6] Stress bio-chemicals also have been linked with delayed wound or surgical healing [7] and heart irregularities.[8]

The body's cells have a multitude of receptor sites. These sites both secrete and store many potent bio-chemicals. Communication can originate in the mind or the body. Not only is there ample evidence of chemical communication, the communication is bi-directional. For example, the immune system has been shown to not only have endorphin receptors on its cells but can also secrete endorphins. In addition, many cells in the brain have endorphin receptors and can secrete endorphins. [9] Research has proven that the "mind" is not just in the brain but exists throughout the body. As Candace Pert, a well-known peptide researcher so eloquently puts it, "Peptides are a constant aqueous solution that makes a continuum of the mind and body."

Continuing to use endorphins as an example, we now can understand that through shifting from an adrenaline state to an endorphin state through the use of imagery, we influence the physiology of our brain and the immune system. Using imagery to consciously shift to an endorphin state, we can shift our mood, increase the ability of the killer T-cells to destroy pre-cancerous cells, and decrease the amount of medication required to control pain. [10]

The endorphin peptide and its opiate receptor represent one of the hundreds of peptides and receptors residing on the surface of all the cells in our body. Endorphin is used here as just one illustration of the mind-body connection. The myth of the mind being disconnected from the body can no longer be believed. What we think, how we feel, the images we hold in our mind, physiological responses and the state of the body are intrinsically entwined. The use of imagery as a complementary approach in health and healing has a real place in the new medical frontier.

Since the focus of this book is on the healing stories of imagery, the complex subject of PNI has been kept as brief as possible. Yet, we include it here because it is important for the reader to have a fundamental understanding of the science that supports imagery in the lived experience. For those who are interested in further exploration, additional PNI resources may be found in the last section of this book.

Section Two:
Sacred Stories From
Many Souls

Cherish your visions and your dreams, as they are the children of your soul, the blueprints of your ultimate achievements.
                                                    ~ Napoleon Hill

Imagery for Personal Growth

The source and center of all man's creative power...is his power of making images, or the power of the imagination.

~ George Bernard Shaw

An Eagle Named "Wind"

By an imagery guide

G eorge called me specifically because he was interested in using Integrative Imagery to work with a symbol. He had recently attended a three-day meditation retreat where he gained a great deal of insight about how his interactions with his wife sabotaged his ability to pursue his dreams. During and after the retreat he came to the realization that he needed a "sea change" in the way he approached his marital relationship and his vision for his personal growth. This would require him to be very aware of not slipping into old patterns that no longer served him. He wanted to have a personal symbol to remind him of his commitment to a new approach. He told me that in the past he had a variety of experiences with guided imagery, imagery incorporating music, and shamanic journeying and was comfortable with the idea of seeking answers within. He had experienced a rich array of sensations when in the imaginal state, with a strong emphasis on the visual.

George got comfortable in his chair and settled easily into progressive muscle relaxation as evidenced by slowed breathing, facial softening, and a quiet, grounded energy. I asked him to invite a symbol to appear that represented for him his new approach to his marriage and his personal goals. I encouraged him to begin describing the image once he had a clear sense of it. He was silent for quite a long time, then began to speak. "It's a bald eagle with a white head. He is strong, big, wise, and has deep vision. He is soaring." I did some sensory recruitment and the experience remained largely visual for him, as he described the eagle's color, the patterns of the feathers, the way the feathers shimmered in the light, and the blue sky. He noticed that every now and then the eagle would open its wings and then come back to a still position. I asked him the image's name. "His name is 'Wind.'" What followed was an interval in which he reported the messages Wind had to share with him. I was struck with the beauty of the words and fortunately he was speaking slowly enough for me to write them down verbatim.

He required very minimal guiding in this portion of the session. An occasional "anything else?" or repetition of a key word was all that was needed to maintain the momentum of the message. When it felt complete, I invited him to ask Wind if there was anything else he needed to say before they said good-bye for now. He described the final message, thanked the image and indicated he was ready to end the session. I guided him slowly back into his body and into the room. He seemed relaxed as he came back to ordinary consciousness. He did not wish to write or draw about the experience, but was interested in talking about it.

George found it easy to articulate the power of this symbol and the essence of the message he had received from it. He was struck for the first time by how the eagle seemed to be a symbol that held importance for him on a number of occasions in his life. Specifically, he spoke of a clay eagle that he made as part of some work he was doing with a therapist during a difficult time early in his adult life. In addition, he remembered that at his wedding, a friend gave him and his wife each a single eagle feather to commemorate their union. He had recently been to Alaska on business and had been planning to go to the eagle nesting grounds nearby. As it turned out, he was unable to fit it into his schedule and had an extremely hard time shaking off his disappointment when he got home. The primary message he brought back from the eagle was to stop trying to control. To hold his goals and vision for himself clearly and trust that if he let go of his need to control his dreams would fall into place for him.

I asked him what he would do with this information. His plan was that each morning before he got out of bed, he would place his hands over his heart, visualize his eagle, and remind himself of his intention to let go and allow his dreams to unfold rather than trying to coerce and control. I asked him if there were any other circumstances when he might want to call forth the image of his eagle. He replied that he thought it would be helpful to turn his attention to a mental image of Wind anytime he noticed himself getting "off track" or getting in the way of creating a smooth marital relationship that was spacious enough to contain the goals they both hold dear. I asked him if he remembered any specific phrases Wind had said. He replied that he really was left more with the essence of the message rather than the exact words.

As in all sessions, I was profoundly aware of this experience as sacred space. It is a privilege to witness another's inner exploration and to be a part of creating the environment to facilitate the process. I did not feel compelled to probe for details about the specific behaviors he wanted to change and how he felt he needed to be in his marriage, or how his wife responds to him when he gets overly controlling, etc. It was evident that he was sharing as much as he needed to and my job was simply to support him in his process - the details are his business. That felt very light and right. The next day, I typed up the words that Wind had said and added a picture of an eagle to the page. I mailed him his poetry and felt like the work was complete. He emailed me when he received the page and told me it was one of the most precious gifts he had ever received.

Wind

Wind is wind because of the power of trusting
the wind,
the power of trusting the universe,
the power of trusting the ebbs and flows of life.

Wind says that you'll never get anywhere if you
fight the wind,
If you're trying to control the wind.

Wind is always changing:
sometimes it's still,
sometimes it's a hurricane.

Wind also says that it's important to open your
wings.
It's important to open your sails and point in
the direction you desire
And at that point it's a matter of trust that the
wind will take you
In the direction you are destined to go.
You'll never get to that destiny if you don't
open your wings and point.
If your wings are shut you ain't gonna get
there.

Wind says that it's so essential to stand in the
vision
To hold the vision
To have perspective
And that the universe will conspire to support

my dreams
If I hold my trust and my faith
And don't try to control things.

Don't run from the dream.
Keep the dream alive every day.
There's no need to control.

A Peaceful Presence

By a student guide

*I*f stress can take its toll physically, my client, Henny, was a prime example. At the time she had two family members and their children staying with her, her husband and their four children. Her physical symptoms came forth as hives on her arms and upper body that appeared during times of stress or tiredness, which she was feeling a lot lately.

In discussing our imagery work, we decided that a session to invite forth an inner healer would be of most help to her now. After doing a surprisingly easy progressive relaxation process, I invited her to form an image of a special place, which for Henny was a beautiful beach in northern California. Cool water was washing up on her feet with warm sand below her. The sky was a beautiful, rich blue and she was alone with the sound of the rhythmic waves. At that point we invited an inner wisdom/ inner healer figure to form in her imagination. Although she could not see him, she described a sensation that was the most powerful and peaceful feeling she ever felt as Jesus made His presence known to her. I noticed that as she described His presence near her, her arms and legs were covered in goose bumps. She said that being with Jesus felt, for her, as a warm bright light that enveloped her entire body.

Henny was quiet for a time, almost as if she were listening. She said Jesus had explained to her that He was always there to take care of her and that she should not worry about the hives or feel stressed or tired. If she prayed when she needed a lift, He would always be there to give it to her.

I asked her how she could bring this feeling inside her when she was feeling the most stressed and she replied, "by praying."

Even before I suggested that she thank this wisdom figure, she spontaneously was thanking Jesus on her own. She spent a few more minutes savoring this moment and then opened her eyes.

Henny looked so relaxed and at peace with herself. She smiled and said, "Can you come and do this for me every day?"

Helping people gain a sense of empowerment over their stressful situations can be so freeing. Often, religious figures that a person is already comfortable with can provide a welcome source for this transformation.

Wrapped in a Blanket of Trust

By a student guide

Marsha is a fifty-year-old married female who works as an accountant in Chicago. She came to the imagery session with a request to work on gaining trust in her relationship with her twenty-year-old son. She explained that when her son was in his early adolescence, he was caught smoking marijuana with his friends. Understandably, it was a very stressful time for the family and since that time she has worried that when he goes out at night, he is still engaging in this behavior. She said that she feels this "mistrust" most when he comes home late at night after being out with his friends. She explains that he usually comes into her bedroom when he gets in to let her know that he is home and it's at this point that she feels tempted to turn on the her light and look in his eyes to see if he's been smoking pot. She resists doing so because she knows that it would infantilize her son. Her husband, who feels more trusting, reminds her that their son was fifteen-years-old when the problem occurred and he is now 20 and has proven himself trustworthy. She said that her lack of trust in her son puts a wedge between them and she worries that if she doesn't find a way to manage it, their relationship will deteriorate.

Marsha was unfamiliar with imagery, so I explained the process to her and suggested that we use a technique called "accessing inner strengths." I explained that this technique involved working with a personal quality or strength, (i.e. trust, courage etc.) that one could call up and draw upon in a challenging situation. I told her that I would ask her to go to a place in her imagination where she felt this specific quality intensely and then, via a cue from this place, transfer it to a second, more challenging situation where she felt she needed the strength of this quality. I explained that during the imagery part of the session, I would ask her to look around to see if she could identify an object, sound etc. that might act as a cue to remind her of this preferred quality. I also introduced her to the idea of amplifying or reducing the intensity of the quality in the situation as needed.

She agreed to give it a try and identified that she would like to possess the quality of "trust" when her son came in late at night. When I asked if she could imagine a situation any time in her life when she experienced intense trust, she quickly described a time in her childhood when she was sitting alone in her bedroom. At this point, Marsha began to cry and apologized for being so emotional. I assured her that emotions often accompany imaging sessions and that what she was experiencing was normal. I suggested she take a few deep breathes and let me know when she was ready to continue. She signaled with a nod that she was ready and I asked if she would be willing to go to this place in her imagination during the imagery session and she said "yes." Then I asked her to identify a specific situation where she would like to have this quality and she said, "In my current bedroom, late at night when my son comes in to tell me he is home."

Because Marsha didn't really know much about relaxation I suggested we start with simple breathing and muscle relaxation and then once relaxed, use a technique called "going to a special place." I started the session by encouraging her to get comfortable on the couch, closing her eyes and then taking a few deep breaths. I suggested that she allow an image to form of a special place and when she arrived there, to describe it. She described a beach where the family went when her children were young. She said that it was early morning and the sun was already hot. She was sitting on a towel in the sand next to her husband and her two boys were playing happily nearby. The air was fresh and the wind was blowing gently so that she could smell the water. She was smiling and stated that she felt "so relaxed". I suggested that she take a couple of deep breaths and then allow an image to form of her childhood bedroom, the one she described as a place where she felt trusting. She quickly described a small room that contained only a bunk bed. She said the light was dim but that she could see the kitchen from where she sat and that the bright lights that illuminated it felt reassuring. After taking some time to feel the trust she experienced in this space, she was ready to look around to see if she could identify something that could act as a cue for this quality. She said that she saw a bed blanket that might work. She described it as a brightly colored striped blanket that looked cozy and warm. In her imagery, she put it around her shoulders for a few moments and took in the pleasure of this sensation of "trusting."

Now that she had "anchored" this feeling of trust by using the image of the blanket around her, she allowed an image to form of her present bedroom when her son comes in late at night to tell her that he's home. She said it was dark in the room and late at night. She heard the front door open and close, which indicated to her that her son was home. She described his presence at her bedside and then said that all of a sudden her body felt "tight." She said she was feeling anxious and wanted to turn on the light to see him. I suggested she take a few breaths and reminded her that if she wanted to, she could use her cue, the striped blanket, to help her gain trust. She was quiet for a while, so I asked how she was doing. She started to cry and said that she would like to put it around him. She then said that instead of imagining putting it around him in this situation, she would picture putting it around him before he leaves to go out at night, with this gesture representing her trust in him. I reminded her about the possibility of amplifying or decreasing the quality and she said that she needed it to be up as high as it could go. She said she felt encouraged by this image and said that she was looking forward to trying it out in real life. I asked if there was anything else and she shook her head. I gently reminded her that it was almost time to end the session and wondered if there was anything else she would like to say or do before we ended. She said that she was feeling gratitude, so I suggested that she might like to thank the images for coming and she smiled and nodded. I then reminded her that it was time to end and suggested that when she was ready, to come back to real time by gently moving her fingers and toes and slowly opening her eyes.

Marsha was very satisfied with the session and afterwards continued to elaborate on how the blanket image could be used. She thought that she could make a point of hugging her son before he went out and while doing so, throw the imaginary blanket around him to protect him in an effort to let go and trust him. She then reconsidered and said that this gesture may be too cumbersome and instead thought she could shrink it and secretly place it on his cheek as she kissed him goodbye before he left to go out at night. She was happy with this alteration and said that she was really looking forward to trying it out. She thanked me and expressed her amazement in the imagery process.

Freeing Trauma from the Past and the Present

By a student guide

I have always loved horses, finding a blend of physical and mental health in being with them. One of my dear friends knew my older horse was nearing the end of his life, so she recently gave me one of her horses. When I was in my Integrative Imagery training, I had to choose a practice session dealing with inner wisdom. I decided to explore with the wise part of myself "why I was clinching up in fear when riding this new horse, named Chili Pepper." Little did I know that I would go on an imagery journey of regression back to a forgotten horse accident I had over 13 years previously. The incident culminated at the edge of a cliff. In the momentum of the jump I had to throw myself off of the horse to avoid being crushed upon landing. In the accident, I dislocated my shoulder. The horse's injury resulted in lameness and an early death. With the imagery experience, I was able to gain the knowledge of how this trauma was affecting not only my bonding with the new horse but also other aspects in my life when I would feel emotions of fear.

In the BON training I was learning to trust the wisdom of the imagery process and honor the sacred space in which to work. The next day, I decided to continue to work on this issue by going back to the event with an inner strength. This is another Integrative Imagery technique whereby one can deal with a current situation by calling for an inner strength from within our experience to use in the present. In the second session, with my guide's assistance, I was able to face the "event" gleaning the knowledge that the new horse, Chili Pepper, had the same habits and head set that the previous horse had demonstrated. As I sat on the cliff in the imagery session, with my inner strength of courage, I was able to counter the feelings of fear and pain. My new horse, even though having similar characteristics to my first horse, was in fact, an individual with his own habits. I was able to turn up my courage, reduce the fear and know that I could move forward with the understanding that I could handle the past trauma in my life with an attitude of a survivor. I now use a cue created in the imagery session of rubbing my fingers together anytime I start to clinch up in fear, knowing I do have the courage to handle fears. Chili Pepper and I have bonded and enjoy riding the foothills of the San Joaquin Valley with the physical and emotional benefits I once had before my trauma event. I am not limited from the trauma of the past but am now free and empowered with the courage to face the challenges life has to offer. I hope this enlightens others to know that we can move beyond our fears.

A Very Special Place

By a student guide

*J*ames is a highly educated man who has never had any experience in simple relaxation techniques or guided imagery.
He would like to be able to relax at any given moment. I explained
to him that imagery is a process in which we use the power of our
minds to gather insight into a particular concern, issue or symptom.
As he had never experienced a relaxation or imagery session, we
discussed how the session would proceed so he would know be-
forehand what to expect. We agreed to do a relaxation process,
then when he felt his body relaxed and comfortable we would begin the imagery by inviting him to create a special safe place in his
mind's eye. This would be a place of beauty, peace and safety
where he felt comfortable and very much at one with nature and
himself. With the agreement in place, we began.

After the initial induction period in which James became very
relaxed and comfortable, I invited him to create a special place in
his mind's eye and said, "Let me know when you are there. This is
your special place. Be open to whatever is here for you."

My client nodded and began to describe his special place. "I
am in one of the pools at Havasupai in the Grand Canyon. It is late
afternoon and the sun is casting a golden shadow on the canyon
walls. The water is warm, smooth, bubbling and noisy. I can move
freely. There is a large waterfall 300 feet away. The rocks are rings
of water pouring from basin to basin. It is very comfortable, very
relaxing. I am very aware of the temperature. It is almost that of
the body. I can move freely in the water without fear. It is a safe
haven: very simple, very complex, very beautiful."

I said, "Say more about that."

James responded, "I feel like I am able to expand beyond my body. The body is the same as the water." (He began to gently weep.)

I paused for a few moments. Then I said, "Stay with it."

A few more minutes passed, so I said, "What are you feeling?"

"I feel one with Nature."

James was quiet for a while.

I asked, "What is happening?"

"I like being in the water. My safe place is by myself. There is only one special pool for me. It is arranged differently than the other pools: it is the right size, shape, and dimension just for me. It is a close experience like being in a womb-- the safety, the warmth, the fit, also the singleness. The waterfall is my mother's heart-beat."

With that my client's eyes opened and he was fully present in the room.

After the imagery experience James took a few moments to ground himself. Then I asked, "Is there anything you would like to share about your experience?"

"That was a very profound experience. It was one of those 'Ah-ha' moments in life. I was so relaxed and comfortable amongst all the pools of water but there was only one particular pool that was the perfect fit and temperature. When I was in the pools of Ha-vasupai in the 1970's I had a similar feeling of being one with the water, but I didn't understand it. Now I do. My safe place was analogous to my mother's womb. The sound of the waterfall was her heartbeat, the perfect fit, the warmth, the perfect temperature. It all makes sense now. Thank you. Thank you."

Blue Shoes

By an imagery practitioner

Stress eating is a life issue for me. I ate potato chips, chocolate and lots of pasta when I felt overwhelmed. These foods calm the chatter of anxiety located in my gut. Nothing like a bag of Lay's chips to make it all OK!

A few years back I decided to go full force to tackle this issue of overeating. I wanted to be in control in this area of my life. The consequences of not being in control were accumulating. I was putting on pounds, my adrenals were very tired and under functioning, I was moody and I just felt plain awful. I was also in perimenopause. My entire being screamed for help. I yearned to have my energy back. My lifestyle had stolen it away. With age, I've learned it's a lot easier to get help with lifestyle changes, so I enlisted the help of a nutritionist. She is a registered nurse who helps people with food issues. My issue was compulsive overeating. She told me I was a food addict. It took me a long time to digest that label and to understand the compulsive nature I had with food.

The nutritionist explained to me in a steady nurturing voice that I was to eliminate caffeine, sugar, dairy and wheat from my food intake. The initial thought in my head was, "you must be crazy, lady." Coffee, croissants, cheese and chocolate were my four basic food groups. I trusted her so I listened even when my mind rejected her wisdom.

I knew she had my best interest at heart.

In the process of getting clean with my food, I began to uncover and discover deep feelings inside my gut. The bag of potato chips was no longer feeding my feelings. I must say I went through a two-month period of severe withdrawal. I got to know the deep anger, hurt and frustration inside my gut for the first time ever. My visceral nerve endings were raw and on fire. Tolerating the un-freezing of feelings in my gut was like living with constant burning embers of coal in my belly region, my power center. This work I was doing with my food was one of the hardest things I've done in my life. The work inside of me was core work, at the center of my being. The old patterns of thinking and ways of being that were no longer useful for me were gasping, clinging to their last breath. I had emotional hunger pains, that called to me all times of the day: "Feed me! Feed me!"

The intensity of the process I was moving through shocked me intellectually. I thought I was so evolved that I was beyond carry-ing anger in my body. I am a seeker and went through years of psychotherapy as well as initiating my own growth and develop-ment. I just couldn't believe the intensity of the anger held in my gut and I wanted it out. Exercise helped some. Eating protein and whole foods helped, too. During this time, light bulbs were blink-ing daily in my head with new messages for me to hear. One con-sistent message that entered my consciousness was "if you use your voice and take up more spiritual space in your world, you won't need to take up so much physical space." I had a deep know-ing this was a truth. I desperately wanted to let go of this anger. I wanted my past to become a reference point in my life, not some-thing that continued to drive my present choices. Another truth that came to me was the only way out of this was to forgive. I wanted to be able to forgive all the past injustices done to me and ones that I'd done to myself.

I began reading about forgiveness. I began praying to God to help me to forgive because I knew I could not do this myself. The anger was keeping me stuck both physically and emotionally. I knew instinctively imagery was my portal to learning to forgive and to removing the fermented anger.

I have lots of experience with imagery both as a clinician and client. I believed in the power of its magic. Accessing inner wis-dom seemed natural. Accessing my images would give me direc-tion and instructions on how to forgive.

So, after coming to this realization that imagery would help me through, I made an appointment one day with an imagery guide. I told her, "I want to transform the anger inside into love and light." This simple request unfolded the following discovery. This imagery is working with parts, the part of me that is filled with anger and the part of me that strongly desires compassion and forgiveness.

Image of my Anger

I felt burning fire searing through the vessels of my body when asked to bring forth an image of my anger. I sensed plaque building in my arteries as the fire of anger spread. A dragon's head appeared through the flames, colorful, intense and somewhat lovely. I sensed warrior energy. Flames were blazing out through the nostrils. Steam pressured itself out of the ears. The bottom half of the dragon was a woman dressed in a blue chiffon dress (blue is my mother's favorite color). The blue dress was set off with a darker blue pair of closed toe high heels. The bottom half of this image wanted to walk away while the head of the dragon wanted to engage in fighting. It is interesting to note that anger and sadness were repressed emotions in my family. I was given the nickname "Groucho Marx" if I showed anger and was told it takes fewer muscles to smile than it does to frown. My nutritionist often told me the fat around my belly had to do with unresolved issues with my mother. Note that the dragon woman was outside of my physical body in relation to space.

I then created an image for Compassion/Forgiveness. Dragon woman was asked to stand in the background to allow space for the second image and she complied.

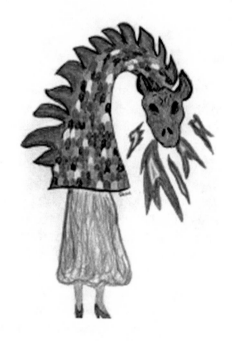

Image of Compassion/Forgiveness

This image came into focus as a flock of butterflies carrying satin ribbons in their mouths. Each butterfly effervescent, almost transparent in hues of pastel gold and glittery sparkles. Each one embraced the qualities of joy, happiness and lightness and was making chirping noises, similar to those of a baby bird. All the butterflies together were playful, free and dancing with ribbon in their mouths. The butterflies were also outside of my body, about arms length away from my heart chakra.

Inviting Anger and Compassion to Have a Conversation

I was asked if the images of anger and compassion would be willing to have a conversation with one another. What unfolded was a large sacred circle with God rays shining to all parts of the circle. I sensed angels were present. There was a fluid white light that focused to a part of the circle like a spotlight.

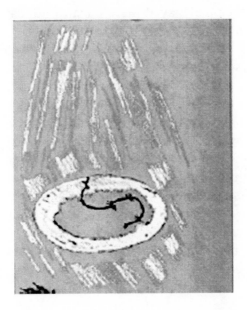

A voice inside of me invited the dragon woman and the butterflies into the circle. The circle was inside of my body now, near the area of my heart. The dragon woman did not want to show up and began shrinking. She held the energy of fear. The butterflies began surrounding the dragon woman, wrapping ribbon around her breath of fire, playfully dancing in-between the breaths of fire. Inside myself I began feeling more calm, stable, and less emotional. The butterflies began chirping in a secret language to the dragon woman, singing to her an invitation to enter the circle and to allow her heart to soften, open and let in the feelings of compassion. The dragon woman and the butterflies entered the liquid spotlight of pure angelic light. The dragon woman melted in the center of the spotlight. Dragon woman's colors then all at once transformed into new butterflies and there were butterflies all over completely filling up the space. The circle transformed into water, angel energy was present and the butterflies were now flying carefree around and over the water that resembled a lake. The color of the lake was a medium blue (like dragon woman's shoes), still and calm without ripples. Green hills appeared surrounding the lake, protecting it. All at once, I felt complete with this imagery experience.

This experience was profound for me. After the session, I left in an altered state and stayed there most of the day. I went home and drew my images. They were breathtakingly beautiful.

As days and weeks passed on I noticed I was able to let go of anger more easily. I was willing to surrender. I held the intention for future anger to move through me rather than take up residence. The anxiety slowly left. My gut was less irritable. I didn't take things so personally. Deep inside my gut I knew healing was beginning. Now when life happens and I get knots of anxiety in my belly, I imagine the butterflies untying the knots, creating long strands of satin ribbon, playful, dancing and creating a sacred space of understanding and compassion inside of me. To solidify this experience I purchased a small statue of Quan Yin, the goddess of compassion. She holds a place of honor in my office. She reminds me to begin my days with an open heart of understanding and love extended to myself and all those who enter my day.

Imagery for Professional Development

First comes thought, then organization of that thought into ideas and plans; then transformation of those plans into reality. The beginning, as you will observe, is the imagination.

~ Napoleon Hill

Transforming the Cage

By a student guide

One of the many benefits of holistic nursing is the necessary focus on self-care as we learn various holistic modalities. Integrative Imagery is a perfect example. The key to becoming proficient in the process is the practice, both as a participant and as a guide. One of the first benefits to a "new" imagery student is the self-knowledge, discovery, and enlightenment that occurs during the process.

My favorite experience occurred when I was practicing conflict resolution imagery. In this exercise you go to a special place and form images for your conflict. My conflict was pretty straightfor-ward-it was my job. I felt I had no control and was being stifled, yet the pay was good; I needed to work; my coworkers and the pa-tients were good; but the hours and workload were always increas-ing.

As I was guided to a special place, I pictured a beach. It was a sunny day and there was a salty smell in the air. I saw in my mind's eye slow breaking large waves that crashed on the shore with a huge spray misting over me. It felt great and I was relaxed.

Once relaxed I was told to form an image for my conflict (sti-fled vs. freedom). I felt trapped in my job, with huge responsibili-ties. The image for my job was a cage with metal bars that were very strong and ugly. I could see out from inside the cage, but it was all around me. Even the door had bars. My other image was a little fairy flying freely wherever she wanted to go. She was beauti-ful, she flew up and down, did back flips, was happy and she was singing. She was radiant-sort of a Tinker Bell type.

When I dialogued with the images, they wanted to be friends.

The cage said it was strong and powerful, dependable and would always be there. It invited the fairy to come in. She said she wanted to be free to do whatever she wanted to, but agreed to fly in. She quickly flew into the cage moving up and around and from top to bottom. As she passed the ugly metal bars, they turned a beautiful, shiny, radiant gold. She giggled as she flew all over, and then the sun from above was shining through the bars so the whole cage was now glimmering. The door was also glimmering and the cage said that it would always be open enough for her to fly in and out as she chose. The cage was very excited about its transformation and was now beautiful as well as strong and dependable. As the images said good by to each other, they vowed to see each other frequently as needed. They would both be there to support each other.

This was a powerful experience for me. I had a new respect for my job. Through the imagery experience I realized that I could be as creative as I wanted to in this job--the door was always open. I was the one thinking I couldn't do what I wanted. I was searching for ways to use complementary modalities in my job, but there weren't enough hours in the day. This was frustrating me. I couldn't find time to conduct patient educational classes or to develop research projects. I was taking holistic nursing courses and couldn't figure out how to incorporate them into my present position. Still, I wanted to stay in the hospital. I wanted to change the cage I had created for myself from ugly metal to a shining radiant gold.

After this experience I began to re-examine my role as a nurse practitioner. I wanted the role to express the qualities of both the fairy and the gold cage: beauty, creativity, freedom, strength, and dependability. I began to develop an outpatient holistic healing series for patients. This three week series addressed healing from a physical, emotional and spiritual perspective and was held after work. I was able to collaborate with the coordinator for patient education to set up the classes, and I was allowed to count the class time as working hours or compensatory time. The patient response to the numerous lectures on imagery, massage, stress reduction and healing was very positive. Also, a research study exploring the effects of touch therapy on nurses was designed, conducted, published and then presented at numerous conferences. All of these accomplishments occurred without changing my job. As the demand for complementary modalities increased, a new nurse practitioner role was created to address patient needs and develop strategies to meet those needs. And guess who took that new job? That's right, it was the little fairy--me.

Being Erin Brockovich

By a student guide

*T*eresa was a client who identified her lack of self-confidence and how it affected her life, especially during interviews for jobs. Teresa wanted to access feelings of confidence as she applied for jobs. The technique was explained very specifically so that Teresa could understand the process. We talked of past imagery she had done, and she stated she was able to visualize in pictures and had some experience with guided imagery. She was not able to identify a time in her life that she felt confident, so she chose a movie character that emulated the quality that she would like to experience. She was also able identify a future situation in which to practice.

The specific feeling she wanted to experience was "self-confidence." The character displaying this quality was the actress Julia Roberts, who played the main character in the movie "Erin Brockovich." She could not specify a scene in the movie but rather some of the gestures and facial expressions of the main character played by the actress. The future situation she wanted to use to practice the feeling of self confidence was "filling out papers for a job."

The office setting was very relaxing without interruptions with soft music playing in the background. After I led Teresa in a head to toe relaxation, I asked her to bring to mind the movie "Erin Brockovich," and allow herself to begin to visualize the actress Julia Roberts and her gestures and facial expressions showing the quality of self-confidence. As Teresa continued in the process her posture started to change. She straightened and sat up more in her chair. Teresa had a difficult time describing her feelings. She stated that it felt good and she also felt happy. She then began to imagine a sprinkler-like fountain originating in her stomach. She worked at increasing and decreasing the intensity of the fountain which, for her, represented the feeling of self-confidence. I used a directive style at this point, stating, "Keeping this feeling, now allow yourself to move to the future situation of filling out the paperwork for a job, taking this feeling with you. Adjust the intensity of this feeling as needed in order to manage this situation with confidence." I kept pace with Teresa and allowed her time to experience this feeling of confidence. I noticed the smile on her face. She used a gesture with her hands to increase the height of the sprinkler. I stated that she could access this feeling anytime and she identified the cue of moving her hands in an uprising gesture to bring this feeling forward. She stated thst she was feeling more relaxed and confident.

Teresa had a chance to share her feelings and said it was a good experience. She stated that she didn't think she would able to make herself feel self-confident and was pleasantly surprised that she was able to do it. She plans to use this gesturing in other areas of her life to increase feelings of self-confidence.

I learned from this imagery session that it's important to trust the process and that it works. As I watched Teresa's posture change and her facial expression broaden into a smile, it made me also smile, as I knew Teresa experienced feelings of low self-esteem and self-worth. In my talks with her following this session, Teresa said it had helped her and that she received feedback from others that she is appearing more confident. Yes!

Creating a New Job with 'Cautious John' and 'Creative John'

By an imagery guide

*J*ohn is a wonderful man who at fifty-four-years-old was seriously contemplating a career change. He had prior experience with the benefits of meditation and imagery and was interested in using imagery once again to assist him in "thinking through" this life decision he was considering. He contacted me and after discussing a little more about the above information, we decided to pursue ways in which Integrative Imagery might assist with his decision.

John had been employed with the same company for 32 years. He had started out in his early twenties sweeping floors and slowly moved "through the ranks" over the years until he held the position of Plant Manager. He spoke of how much he enjoyed his work and how he felt pride in "his plant." He knew the buildings and property he cared for intimately; underground pipes, roof leaks, wall structure, bottling machinery, all he cared for like a loving father. But recently the company had changed hands and the new owners had very different business goals. John found his ideas were cast aside, needed repairs were ignored, and the pride of a "job well done" had vanished from his routine.

John was a talented man. He had always enjoyed fixing and rebuilding things. As a younger man he had built his own home from the ground up. He repaired vintage stoves, cars, children's toys, and one of his favorites – old clocks. He described his home as "Gepetto's Workshop"...filled with chiming, bonging clocks in various states of repair. John was now considering resigning from his job of so many years and opening up a clock repair business in his own home. He spoke of being afraid to leave the security of "a pay check" and despite his obvious talents, "maybe not being good enough at this" to give it a try. Naturally, finances were also a concern. John and his wife had been able to pay off the mortgage to their home recently and the last of their 5 children was in her second year of college. He felt the largest of his financial demands was behind him.

We discussed his previous experience with meditation and imagery. He had been introduced to relaxation and meditation years before while seeing a counselor. He found it extremely helpful at the time, and was hopeful he could use imagery in approaching his current situation and decision. We discussed this type of imagery and I explained that imagery was a form of directed daydreaming where the guide merely assists the individual to become more aware of his own inner reality. We spoke of the inner wisdom present in all of us and he aligned "inner wisdom" with "gut feeling." John acknowledged his desire to find the confidence he felt he once had in himself and in his ability to do things. His fear was that he wasn't good enough...and that this fear might cause him to fail. At the same time, he knew somewhere in himself he could trust his instinct and would succeed! WOW! I was excited to work with John and my head spun with possible techniques...Inner Wisdom, Inner Strengths, Parts Work, and Working with an Image...where to begin? We actually started off slowly, doing a simple imagery technique "Special Place" during our first session. John enjoyed the session, and felt very positive that imagery would be a useful tool for him at this point in his life. We agreed to meet twice a week for the next two weeks, moving from Special Place imagery to Inner Strengths and Parts Work.

The next time we met, John was pleased that he had contacted his 401K retirement program and found that he could, if necessary, make monthly withdrawals from his retirement fund starting with his 55th birthday. This was comforting to him, as he knew it was a financial cushion should it be necessary. We moved to working with Inner Strengths and John remembered how self-assured he was years before when he built his first home. He felt the excitement and energy of planning and building and watching his dream take form. "I could do anything! I wasn't afraid of failure." John felt his self-confidence had been whittled away slowly over the years, and he worked hard to bring this remembered excitement and confidence to his current self. He modulated his feelings by using a hammer and bell, swinging the hammer hard enough to ring the bell at the top of his imaginary pole. He swung--the bell sounded. He likened the bell to the chime of clocks. He was smiling and laughing and so was I! He "anchored" this feeling of rediscovered confidence with an image of his leather carpenter's belt with well used tools hanging comfortably around his waist. John felt empowered by the work of these two sessions, and reported that the feeling did not fade away in the days to come.

The next week, according to our contract, we used the technique of Parts Work. In imagery, John met two parts of himself – a Creative John and a Cautious John. Creative John related experiences in the past that illustrated he was a clever and creative man. He had drafted his own house plans on two occasions. He had worked together with a carpenter he hired and together they built the house he had designed. Creative John was confident in his abilities and was excited about the potential of starting a new business. Cautious John reminded his counterpart that it had been many years since he had designed and built a house. How did he (Creative John) know he still had what it would take to be an entrepreneur? In his current position he received an excellent salary with benefits; he certainly was going to loose that security! He had worked for his employer for over 30 years and his identity was one of "expert" on company property and buildings. He was well known and well liked within his industry. Cautious John remembered and highly respected Creative John; however he felt *he* had the voice of maturity and experience. Creative John likewise respected Cautious John and acknowledged that the *secure* position would be to continue with his current employment, as frustrating and unfulfilling as it had become in recent years.

When John arrived for our second and last session using Parts Work, he shared that it had been an especially frustrating week at work. During the imagery session Creative John was quick to express that he was feeling suffocated by what he perceived as negativism toward John's suggestions for plant improvement. He felt the atmosphere was becoming unhealthy. Cautious John hesitated only slightly and agreed that despite the risk and assured loss of income, it was time to seriously consider leaving. Both "parts" acknowledged that leaving would be best for John. Creative John and Cautious John came together and agreed – starting a private business in fine clock repair would be a challenge, but with careful planning and realistic goals – it could be done! Both parts of John's imagery decided to anchor the feeling of self-assurance with the imaginary tool belt...he would wear it the day he chose to inform his life long employer of his planned "retirement." Two weeks later, with invisible tool belt hanging from his waist, John spoke with his employer and shared his plan of starting his own business. He later said the conversation went very well, and he never faltered in his own conviction that this *was* the right thing to do...for himself and for the company.

Two months later John, business friends and colleagues enjoyed his "retirement" party, given by his long time employer. The following Monday, his clock repair business opened, cautiously, out of John's garage!

One year later John is very busy, with an average of 10 or more clocks at a time on his repair shelf. He certainly has discovered the challenges of owning a small business, but he continues to solve each challenge with cautious creativity! Now he imagines a small storefront window filled with beautiful, old clocks looking for a new home.

After two years of living his vision, John has a year waiting list for his expert clock repair.

To Be or Not To Be,....

Famous

By a student guide

*C*orry is a published author who is in the process of writing another book. She is familiar with imagery and would like to explore the conflict she has about the possibility of being famous and how that would impact her life. The two aspects of this issue that we chose to explore were the conflict between being famous versus non-famous. We discussed relaxation methods and she is comfortable relaxing herself. She wanted to go to a "special place" to begin our session.

I held silent space while my client facilitated her own relaxation. When she reached a comfortable place, she nodded and I began:

"Allow yourself to go to a special, safe, beautiful place, a place you have been before or one you have created in your imagination and when you are there begin to describe what you sense: see.....hear.....smell...feel."

"I am in a beautiful rose garden with a trellis of pink roses. The smell of roses is intoxicating. I am sitting on a marble bench looking through arches to the green mountain beyond. "

"What else are you sensing?"

"I feel so, so ....relaxed here. The sun is warm on my face."

"Take a moment to really enjoy this relaxed special place in the rose garden and when you are ready, allow yourself to invite an image to form that represents the part of you that may be famous."

"She is an Indian. She is a wise, old medicine woman. She is holding a fawn skin medicine bag with turquoise beads hanging from it. She is calm, self-confident and so, so wise."

"What would she like to be called?"

"Her name is Owl Woman."

"What does she want?"

"She wants me to walk down the path with her."

"Go ahead if you like. What does she have to offer?"

"I am walking with her. She is offering me wisdom and trust. She says, "To trust I know the way."

"Now invite the image to appear that represents the part of you that may not be famous."

"It is an old humpbacked Chinese man. He is missing his teeth. He is hunched up. He seems scared and fearful."

"Does the Chinese man have a name?"

"Mr. Yi."

"What does he want?"

"He wants to tell me he is scared. He is scared of the road ahead. He doesn't want anyone to look at him."

"What does he need?"

"To be left alone--to starve, because he has no teeth."

"What does he have to offer you?"

"Only fear and starvation."

"What does Owl Woman feel about Mr. Yi?

"Owl Woman says that she feels love for Mr. Yi and there's nothing to fear but fear itself."

"Let Mr. Yi know that and let Mr. Yi respond."

"Mr. Yi says, 'Easy for her to say, she has teeth.'"

"How does Mr. Yi feel about Owl Woman?"

"Mr. Yi says he admires Owl Woman."

"Let Owl Woman know that and let Owl Woman respond."

"Owl Woman says, "Thank you.""

"Do they have anything in common?"

"Yes, they are on the same road."

"What do they need from each other? "

"They need to trust each other."

"Is there anything that they want to share with each other?"

"Yes. Owl Woman has opened her medicine bag. She pulled

out a lapis bowl and she is filling it with warm broth. She hands it to Mr. Yi and tells him to drink!"

A few minutes went by...

"Tell me more - are they willing to work together?"

"Yes. Mr. Yi is drinking the warm broth. His starvation is going away. He is not as frightened. He trusts Owl Woman."

"What's the next step?"

"Owl Woman has taken Mr. Yi's hand and they are walking down the path together."

"Allow yourself time to thank the images for coming to you. When you are done, gently bring yourself back, remembering what's important to you about this experience."

When the session had ended I asked Corry how she was feeling, what insights she had and if this helped her with her goal. She said she felt much relief. When asked how she planned to integrate this in her life she stated that she planned to continue to write and not worry about how being famous might impact her life. She felt more calm and self-confident.

Embracing the Fire

By an imagery practitioner

Always in the middle of many things in those days, I had taken a red-eye flight to the East coast to participate in the last phase of my imagery certification program. Despite the wondrous intensity of the experiences in the previous phases, I naively expected to squeeze in this last phase and fly back home. I was delighted by the New England charm, the clean fresh autumn air, and, most especially, by the wonderful warm welcome from a group that completed the previous phases together and had never met me. I was embraced by these fellow imagers and learned things about myself from this group that I would have never expected. What I learned has served me well and it carried me through the next several years. In fact, many aspects of that trip nearly seven years ago continue to hold much power for me and those aspects all started so simply.

Our task during this particular phase of the program was to experience imagery about "purpose." It was one of the last experiences in the certificate program, and I already felt pretty clear about the concept of purpose. I was on a path and, in fact, I was intensely engaged with being on that path. So I didn't expect what came next, or what came in the next several months.

Sitting in a simple dormitory style room, my imagery guide invited me to imagine being in my special place with my inner wisdom image, and then to invite an image of my purpose. After some conscious breathing and with the relaxing voice of my imagery guide, I found myself in a familiar alpine meadow surrounded by tall trees. The feel of the dark green grass on my bare feet, the sound of a small nearby stream and the gentle wind whispering in the tall pines, the smell of the rich brown earth, and the strong yet gentle, loving presence of my teacher, "grandmother," and healer (names for my inner wisdom image) all embraced me and immediately put me at ease, at peace, and in knowing. A very familiar and dear animal ally was there as well and contact with this animal, stroking its coat, hearing its breath so close to me, feeling its nudges on me, allowed me to feel completely cared for in a way that I had rarely experienced. This was "home" for me-a place and feeling I had come to know through imagery. After some moments of taking in the love and nurturing there for me, I invited another image. The image of purpose that arose was a ball of intense fire and flames just in front of me. I knew not to be afraid and I knew that the actual image of purpose was to recreate, through my mothering and my teaching and healing work, that very special place with my teacher and animal ally. In that instant, I also knew that the flames were the fire of passion. Passion was the other necessary ingredient for my purpose. The flames entered me through my root chakra at the base of my spine in what can be called a Kundalini experience. I was infused with the flames and a new raw and almost sexual energy, a driving force. As I began to feel this new energy, I realized its power. There was a dizzying, ungrounded quality to this energy, a kind of whirlwind inside. In imagery, so much can happen in less than a nanosecond. That whirlwind was completely unbalancing. I knew not to be afraid, and I knew that, as I later wrote in my journal, "I would have to get used to this." I would have to learn to ground this energy or become completely unbalanced by so much passion. I began working on grounding and I found myself lying on the grass by the stream in the meadow with my teacher and animal ally nearby. I was being tended as I worked on grounding by my teacher, by contact with the rich, brown earth, by the sound of the water, and by grounding itself. My animal ally sometimes exhibits a sense of humor and it rolled its eyes at me and wordlessly communicated, "Here we go again!" This same animal had previously reminded me that some people run animals to death so I became aware that I had to do my best to take good care of myself, thereby caring as well for my animal ally. As before, all of this information and knowing transpired in a flash. It seemed too soon, but my imagery guide was calling me back to the time and space of the room and I gave great thanks to my teacher and animal ally for this completely new energy and relationship with purpose.

It was somewhat challenging to communicate what had just happened and to carry this new energy in a grounded way, especially as I walked out of the room. I knew something very important had taken place and I had no idea what I would do with it. As often is the case, the situation directed me and I found what to do with that energy, at least for the moment. After walking a labyrinth on the grounds of the facility I led the group in a Tree of Life grounding meditation. It was my contribution to the closing ceremony and the perfect way to move forward with this new energy. Again, something so simple can be so powerful.

Perhaps the most important part of the story is what came after that trip, some of which I remember and some of which comes from my journals because things moved very quickly. Within a month and a half, I had co-written a major training grant that created a new curriculum on integrating complementary healing in primary care. The grant was later funded and I was one of the proud birth mothers of the new program. Within two months, I had traveled twice to study other types of healing (rather unusual for me) and continued my full time faculty position and part time nursing practice while single parenting my two daughters. By eight months after the imagery session I had done six professional presentations, three of which were national presentations involving travel. I had co-written a book chapter, and had passed another sixteen units of the graduate program I was working on completing. The driving force of that energy propelled me through more personal changes and healing work; through challenges in parenting my children; through developing a new program and working with my co-workers and graduate students; and through my own graduate program in another field. It wasn't always smooth. As the grant writing finished after many weeks of twenty-hour days, I was hit by a nasty case of vertigo that was rather like that whirl-wind I experienced in the imagery session on purpose. On the morning the vertigo struck me, as I began a slow fall to the floor, the image of my animal ally telling me that some people run animals to death popped into my awareness. Of course, it was time to work on more grounding.

Knowing myself as I do and knowing how it is to have in some way "lost" much of that driving force, at least for this moment in my life, I can say with certainty there is no possible way I could have done what I did without that imagery experience. Was it imagery? Was it shamanic journey? Or was it energy healing? I was certainly well engaged in all three, both doing and receiving, and my experience would meet criteria for all of them. Perhaps part of the beauty of imagery is that it can be all of those and more. As is usual for the imagery program I received far, far more than just the content.

Sometimes an individual has a numinous moment in their life and will hold it in a treasured place in their heart. I feel blessed to cherish many of those moments and I feel doubly blessed to have experienced the far-reaching fruit of one of those life-changing moments.

Imagery for Childbirth

The possible's slow fuse is lit by the imagination.

~ Emily Dickinson

The Littlest Angel

By an imagery guide

*I*n 1996 my best friend, Kelly, was trying to get pregnant. She was not having much success and feeling very sad about her difficulty. One evening she and another friend, Darlene, were over for a girl's night sleepover. During the evening I did a relaxation exercise with them and then suggested to Kelly that she lie down while we played some special music and that she visualize finding her perfect child. We played the CD "Music of the Angels" - specifically a cut entitled "The Playful Ones." Afterward Kelly just wanted to go to bed and sleep. As Kelly slept peacefully, dreaming about her perfect baby, Darlene and I were outside on my patio watching an incredible heavenly event, a comet trailing across the night skies. The next morning when we asked Kelly about her visualization she was very excited as she described her imagery. She told us she found herself in a very beautiful garden that was filled with babies and small children. While in the garden, she encountered a lovely little girl with bright blond hair and beautiful eyes, who came running toward her. She "knew" she had found her baby. Several months later Kelly was indeed pregnant, and very happy.

Before Christmas of that year, Kelly and I were in San Francisco for our annual holiday shopping weekend. Kelly was about four months away from delivery and knew she would be having a girl. However, she was struggling with whether to name the baby Sydney or Taylor. As is our custom, we walked everywhere in San Francisco. What we soon discovered, was that each time we came to an area we were unfamiliar with, and we would look to see what street we were near, we *always* ended up on Taylor Street. This occurred all weekend, and in a variety of areas around San Francisco. At one point, after climbing a very large hill, and emerging from a beautiful garden area between two streets, one of them Taylor Street, Kelly looked up into the sunny blue sky and cried out, "Okay, okay, so I will name you Taylor!" On March 31, 1997, Taylor arrived. She was a beautiful blond haired, brown-eyed, precocious little soul.

In the summer of 1999, when Taylor was two years old, the three of us were enjoying my backyard garden while listening to music. Kelly and I had often discussed putting on the CD we played the night she did her imagery to see if Taylor would have any response to it. Taylor was engrossed in running around the garden, picking posies while shrieking, laughing and playing in the water fountain. After a while the music changed and the Angel song came on. Immediately, there was a shift in Taylor's verbal and non-verbal behavior. She became very quiet, her face softened and she calmly walked over to her mommy, climbed up into her lap, held her hand and cuddled in close, stroking the skin on her mommy's face and hands. When she heard the laughter of the children in the music she perked up and started looking around the yard. She asked, "Where are they?" but she remained closely held in Kelly's embrace. As soon as the music was over she returned to her pre-music persona, jumped off Kelly's lap, looked around the yard and then stated very matter-of-factly, "Well, the kids are gone now!" Kelly and I were struck by the unmistakable change we had witnessed. We asked Taylor who the kids were and she said, "They are the babies in the garden." We had no doubts that Taylor had connected with the music.

A few months passed and Kelly and Taylor were visiting again and we were in my home office listening to music. We put on the Angel song once more and Taylor became quiet, wanted to sit on Kelly's lap and this time talked about the babies in the angel garden when she heard the laughter of the children in the song. Kelly then asked Taylor to tell me about who she was talking to in her bedroom the day before their visit. She looked at me with those "old soul" eyes and proudly told me that she was talking to the angels that were in her room.

In mid-2001 Kelly and Taylor moved to North Carolina. Although we see them infrequently we all remain very spiritually connected. When my husband and I went to visit in late 2001 Kelly waited to tell Taylor until the night before we arrived. Taylor immediately went to her room and dug out of her immense toy chest a small pink bear I had given to Kelly when she delivered Taylor. Taylor brought it down to Kelly and said, "Look what I found, this has always been my favorite bear." Kelly asked her if she knew who gave her the bear and Taylor did not. When Kelly told her I had given it to her at her birth she just laughed. Taylor carried that bear around the entire week we visited them.

Our worlds are only a veil apart, and it is so wonderful to have Taylor in our lives, allowing us to peer through that veil still. Kelly and I have no doubt whatsoever, that on that night in 1996, while doing a very powerful imagery, she traveled to the angel's baby garden and found her perfect child. Seeing and hearing Taylor's perceptions are true blessings and reminders that we exist on many levels.

A Mom Ready for Her Twins

By an imagery guide

Susan, my client who was pregnant with twins, asked for guided imagery to help her with the induction of labor the following day. I took time to explore what exactly she wanted help with and she said she had anxiety and found it difficult to trust. She said she had been watching the annual Roe V. Wade discussions. One woman was passionately telling that she had had an abortion and when she went into labor with her next child, she had a long difficult labor. Susan had had an abortion many years before. We talked about her labor with her living son, and it had been a 12-hour labor. In open, clear, and gentle language, we talked about several different perspectives on what she was saying. We talked a bit about the uterus and how miraculously it does its work. Then I suggested using a choice of imagery techniques: "working with an image;" "inner wisdom;" or "inner strength." She had used "inner wisdom" in the past and wanted to try "inner strength." She also wanted to take time to create the safe and comfortable place and experience relaxation. She and I agreed on how we would proceed: she wanted to see if a combination of working with an image and inner strength might work. She said she would take a rubber ball she had with her to labor and use that as the anchor. We also discussed the times she felt the most joyful and relaxed.

Susan lay on her left side and I facilitated her relaxation and breathing, to encourage a relaxed state. Next we went to her special place - a Disney beach with her husband and son. She formed a very clear image of when she was relaxed, calm, happy, loving and fulfilled. Her heart was full. She experienced no pain or discomfort. Using the "intensity scale" to increase these good feelings, she easily imagined a dial and turned it up a notch to a 7 on a 0-10 scale. Then when she turned the imaginary dial down a few notches she saw herself in a hospital room. She turned it back up and she was hearing children playing on the beach and her husband splashing with her son. She was very content.

Next we imagined her labor and Susan used both breathing and the modulating dial to "practice labor." She also saw her cervix opening like a camera lens and she could see both of the boy twins peeking out of one of those toy expandable tunnels. I asked what the twins wanted to say and she said they were just giggling. I asked what this meant to her and she said she knew they were happy and healthy and just about ready to come out to the world. I asked if she wanted to say anything to them and she told them she would wait for them, but if they would come out, she had some ice cream for them. They were all laughing. I suggested she tell them it was safe and that they will be loved.

We then went back to imagining her labor and she talked to her uterus and envisioned herself in a hammock just swaying back and forth. Each time she swayed her cervix opened a bit more. She loved this image and incorporated it into her beach scene. The twin boys chose which one would come first and told her it was very important. They agreed they would come without reluctance. Her uterus said it was ready and able to do its work and she could clearly see the delivery of both babies with everyone smiling and even joking. We anchored the feeling of joy, peacefulness, and relaxation on the beach with her squeezing the small rubber ball. She used the dial when she wanted to amplify the feeling of calm. She would tune into the sound of the waves and the feeling of the swaying hammock with each contraction. She was now clear and calm, so we gently ended the session.

When we discussed what had happened in this session, Susan was very excited and confident. She remembered the scale with the dial and the anchoring using the rubber ball. She was amazed and loved the images and feelings she experienced. Susan truly believed she would use them the following day. She invited me to check in with her tomorrow. She left smiling, relaxed and filled with a sense of quiet expectation.

The next day I checked in with her when she was beginning labor. She was smiling and already using the imagery. I gave her a relaxation session with her husband present and we used her images from the day before. She was comfortable at that time. When I checked with her after the birth she said the labor was about eight hours from the time she started contractions and that she was thrilled with how it went. The babies are beautiful!

Imagery in Living and Dying

Imagination is evidence of the divine.

~ William Blake

With Help from the Choir

By an imagery guide

*O*ne of the reasons Integrative Imagery is so powerful is that clients choose their own healing path under the guidance and gentle direction of a guide. This story is about this aspect, and also about how surrendering to the process that is occurring *with* the client and *between* the client and the guide allows healing to occur and allows magic to happen!

One of the places I do imagery and other healing work is in a clinic at a church in the city I live in. The church is located in the heart of the city, in an area frequented for many years by addicts, prostitutes, homeless, mentally ill and disabled people and in recent years, many Southeast Asian immigrant families. This church is known for its charismatic minister who has embraced all these folks and many call this church their home—they are fed here and get help with many social services including recovery programs, job training, and health care. The church is also known for its spirited Sunday services with a wonderful multi-racial gospel-style choir and live band. People from all walks of life and socioeconomic status attend these services and belong to the church. The health clinic offers basic medical care but also is unique in providing, at no cost, various complementary healing services such as imagery, energy healing, acupuncture, chiropractic, and massage.

"Diane," a parishioner, dropped by the clinic one morning hoping to get an appointment with the acupuncturist. A tall, poised, neatly dressed woman with short gray hair, she informed me she was in the midst of receiving chemotherapy for stage IV lung cancer and wanted help with the side effects of chemo, specifically the feelings of numbness and tingling in her feet and lower legs.

The acupuncturist was fully booked that day, but I had an opening and so we began a therapeutic relationship that lasted several months. Our initial sessions dealt with finding ways for her to decrease these uncomfortable feelings in her legs and feet. In our first session she decided she wanted to access an inner healer, and her Reiki (an energy therapy) teacher appeared and began working on her feet. Diane told me later that she used this image over and over again to soothe her pain.

One day, after having not seen Diane for a couple of months, she came to the clinic and told me that the cancer was metastasizing in other parts of her lungs. For the first time, she wanted to have an imagery session focused on the actual cancer, in particular, the metastasis in her lungs. We decided to do a session in which she would create an image that represented the new cancer tumor in her right lung and interact with this image in the hopes of gaining information for her healing.

After guiding her into a relaxed state, I asked her to request an image of the tumor in her right lung to appear. This image was a large sticky mass. I suggested to Diane that she describe the mass' qualities, but it started to grow and she started becoming frightened.

I suggested she ask it what it wanted, but the image would not speak, it would only expand and spread, like a huge messy gummy mass on the floor. As it grew it became more and more intimidating. Diane was frightened, and I was about to panic—what had I done? Thoughts raced through my mind such as, "Why did I try to venture into such risky territory?" "Yikes! I don't know what to do!" "I must save her!"

But luckily, the voices of my imagery teachers came through, stating, "Trust the process." I took a deep breath, centered, and asked Diane if there was anyone or anything she wanted to be there with her to help her. There was a long pause. Then she said, "Oh! The Reverend is here! He is helping me mop up this mess." There was a brief silence, and then, "Oh! The choir is also here and they are singing...and the whole congregation is here too! They're singing 'Wade in the Water,' and everyone is mopping. It is such hard work and it is going slowly, but they are all helping me with this. They are scrubbing and scrubbing and singing." Tears rolled down her face.

At this point, as the guide, I could only hold the space for this work to unfold, and feel humbled and honored to be a part of this sacred process.

This kind of thing has happened over and over again in imagery sessions in which I have facilitated, and it always surprises me and puts me in awe of the power of the body's self-healing abilities.

Diane passed away about a year or so after the above session. However, some months before her death she told the clinic director that our imagery sessions helped give her a sense of control even in the face of a terminal illness. For this client, healing did not mean curing her illness—we both understood this wasn't going to happen through our sessions. The healing that occurred in these imagery sessions was about accessing inner strength and resources that allowed her to feel stronger and less alone in her final journey.

Being Brave Enough to Offer

By a student guide

*O*ne day, on the cardiology unit where I work, I had a patient, "Len," who I dreaded working with after hearing report from the other nurses. He had inoperable lung cancer and was currently on hospice care, but had been brought to the hospital with rapid heart beat and chest pain, as well as nausea and vomiting. I looked at his heart rhythm on the monitor and what I saw concerned me. As soon as I met Len I was struck by his anxiety and quiet despair. He was only in his late fifties, but looked haggard and weak as an old man. I asked him if he would like a session of Integrative Imagery a little later in the afternoon, if he felt up to it. I described what imagery is and how it works, and he said he was interested. I let him sleep for a few hours as doctors discussed his doubtful case.

Because of the business at work that day, I went to Len's room after the shift was over and I had time to devote to Len. I asked the new shift nurse to give us twenty minutes before she came to assess him, so we would have a little privacy in a not-very-private setting. Len said he would still like a session when I checked in with him. He was tired, but alert. I began with a head-to-toe relaxation with him and he settled more deeply into his pillows, breathing easily. I directed him to imagine a special healing place, and when he was comfortable there, to ask for an image of his Inner Healer to appear. "The inner healer is one who is wise and loving and knows just what you need to heal, and can help you," I explained. I sat silently and waited for at least five minutes, and was just about to leave the room, concerned that he had fallen asleep in the relaxation. Suddenly he spoke. "It's Jesus," he said. I was a bit surprised and shocked at his sudden words, but I recovered and asked him to describe Jesus. "He's about five foot ten, 170 pounds." I asked, "And what is He wearing?" He described flowing blue robes and a golden aura around the image's head. "Is this the image of the Inner Healer you want to work with now?" "Yes," Len replied. "Is there something you would like to ask Jesus?" Len began to weep and said, "I want to ask Him to let me live. I don't want to die. I'm not ready to die!" "Go ahead and tell him that," I said. There was a pause in which he continued to cry quietly. "What's happening now?" "Jesus is holding me and telling me it's alright. He says I will be fine, if I stay with Him." "Is there anything else you would like to convey to Jesus?" Len started sobbing then, and said, "I want to thank Him for my life, for my kids and especially for my wife. She's been with me for 35 wonderful years and she is so good to me. Thank you, Jesus!" He kept crying, and after a time I said, "Take a few moments to take whatever else you need from the image, remembering that Jesus is always with you as your Inner Healer and you can be with Him any time you want. Then thank Him for coming, and when you are ready, come back to this time and place."

When Len opened his eyes, he reached for my hand and we sat for a few minutes while he spoke about how much the session had meant to him. He said he felt much better about things, and he would tell his wife how much he loved her. I reminded him that he could bring the image back whenever he needed his Inner Healer, and thanked him for the session.

I had the next day off, but when I came in to work the day after, I learned that Len had two cardiac arrests and had died in the ICU. I was upset to hear this, but I was very glad that I had done an imagery session with him when I did. Of course I will never know, but I would like to think that the transition between life and death was somewhat eased for Len because of his meeting with his inner healer. I learned from this experience that when one has the intuition that it is appropriate to offer an imagery session, to go ahead and *do it then*.

Grief Can be Bearable

By a student guide

Lisa was dealing with the impending death of her husband. She was already experiencing grief and came to me looking for healing work in that regard. We had a conversation about guided imagery, which she had used in the past. I asked which image she wished to use: "wisdom figure;" "inner strength;" or "inner healer" as possible ways to approach the issue. She decided to ask for her inner healer to help her with emotional healing. She was weary from taking care of her sick husband but calm. Her physical health was good although she had been in an automobile accident earlier in the year and had hurt her neck. Her spiritual belief system was eclectic including parts of Christianity, Native American, Buddhism, and was connected to nature. She was comfortable with metaphor and meditates daily. Her means of relaxation was through breathing.

As soon as Lisa had used deep breathing to relax, in her mind's eye she went to her cabin up north. She described the place in detail including mid-afternoon light, smelling the pines, feeling the dampness, hearing the loons and the water lapping against the rocks. She began to cry. I asked her how she felt with the tears and she said she was afraid. I asked her what she noticed about the fear and she said she feared death. She was afraid of her husband dying-supporting him in the process, being present for it, his discomfort, the unknown, her own loneliness and loss of a spiritual partner. I allowed her to feel her feelings for a while and then asked her to become more comfortable there in her imaginary cabin. She moved to a rocking chair and I asked her to let herself relax and let comfort wash over her. She visibly relaxed and grew quiet. I suggested she invite an image of an inner healer (someone or something that was wise, loving, compassionate and strong and knew exactly what she needed today) to come to her mind's eye. Instantly she saw a black bear come ambling toward her outside the cabin. She felt a warmth and comfort right away. The bear had a lighter snout and dark eyes. It was about four feet tall. I directed her to greet the bear in whatever way was comfortable for her. I asked, "Is the bear your inner healer?"

"Yes."

"Ask the bear why it is here today."

Lisa said that the bear was there to help her with her grief and fear.

"How will she do that?"

"She wants to talk with me."

Lisa was quiet for a bit and then I asked what was happening and she said she had explained to the bear how sad she feels losing such a good friend. Tears come so easily these days. And now there is fear attached as well.

"What will the bear do?"

"She'll sit there with me. Support me. Hold me. Teach me a few things about soft, warm, fuzzy, and loving."

"Is there anything you want to ask the bear?"

"I would like her to show me the cause of the grief. The bear says it's the loss of things and about changes. It's all about birth and death and letting go. Letting go of the things we love is hard and there will be grief. But she'll teach me more about it and about having some fun too. She also says that my husband will be fine and will help to take care of me too."

"Is there anything else?"

"No."

"Before we close, ask how you can get back in contact with her for further work."

"The bear says all I have to do is pull on my right ear like Carol Burnett as a signal for her presence."

A thank you was said and the image of the bear faded. The client gradually returned to an alert state.

Lisa took a minute to readjust and began to smile. She was relaxed and visibly lighter.

I asked her what she remembered about the experience and she said the warmth of the bear. And that she felt comforted by the nurturing energy of the bear. I asked her to sit with that feeling and to let it integrate by allowing the feeling to wash over her. When I asked if she was able to recall the feeling she said yes.

"Did this imagery experience give you any insights?"

"Yes, I really liked the cycles of life piece." She felt tenderness and strength. She was also relieved that she would have fun again in her life. The most fun she had in her life has been with this man who has been in her life for only four years. In the future, she will call on the bear by pulling on her ear and she can spend time during meditation seeking the bear's comfort and solace. We laughed about the pulling of the ear. She paused a moment and then said, "I couldn't have ever made this up!"

Our Lady of Guadalupe Claims Her Own

By an imagery guide

A s a psycho-spiritual counselor in a large cancer practice I had the opportunity to work with many clients who were facing their death. It is always a difficult topic to discuss with clients. Through many trial and error sessions I became experienced at letting clients know I was someone who was safe to discuss these issues with and at the same time I was someone who would not push them to discuss it until they were ready.

Jimmy was a Hispanic man who, with his wife, attended my cancer support group for seven months. He did not speak of his issues very much during the group but was very attentive and quick to give a word of encouragement to the other members. During that time his colon cancer had proved resistant to treatment and he had become progressively more debilitated until he ended up in the hospital. He had very good family support from his second wife, Sandy, and his adult daughter from his prior marriage.

When I came to visit Jimmy in the hospital he was quite agitated and concerned that he was not going to ever get out of the hospital, in other words, that he was going to die there. I mentioned that we had not really discussed the topic of his death and wondered if he would like to do that.

Jimmy immediately became very tearful and upset. He said that he and his wife now attended a Methodist church but that he had been raised Roman Catholic. He stated he was very afraid he would be going to hell because he was divorced. Sandy and he had not been married in the Roman Catholic Church because of the divorce. He was very concerned that all of the worst stories of death and after life would come true in his case.

Guided imagery is often a way to help clients get to the heart of matters quickly and I hoped that Jimmy would be able to revise the picture of his death to one that would give him more peace of mind. I asked him if he felt willing to do some imagery that would help him understand what would be a healthy and peaceful death for him. He said, "It sounds pretty crazy to me, but since I have known you all those months in the group I think I can trust you."

After helping Jimmy relax and find an inner-focused place, I asked him to imagine a time when he felt confident that he was loved by God. He quickly described a time that occurred frequently throughout his childhood. The local church of the small town in Southern California where he was raised had a niche on one side where there was a statue of the Virgin of Guadalupe. He smiled as he described the special love he had for the Virgin and how he would often go to sit beneath Her and speak of his hopes and dreams. He enjoyed several moments of the imagery session re-experiencing the love and support he felt from Her. His face, which had reflected discomfort and agitation, became softer and much more relaxed. I asked him if there were any questions that he wanted to ask. He asked several questions about his life, but he did not ask Her any questions related to his death. I suggested that he tell Guadalupe about this situation concerning his divorce and remarriage. At first his face tensed and then relaxed again. He poured out the whole story to Her. When I asked him how She responded to the story, he smiled and said, "She still loves me, and She is proud of me that I learned lessons from my first marriage and worked so hard to make my second marriage happy." I asked if there was any thing else, and he said, "I want to ask Her if I will go to heaven, despite what the church says, but I am afraid." I suggested that he look into the face of the image and see if it felt safe to ask. He said it did, so he asked. After a series of emotions passed across his face, he finally relaxed and said, "She tells me that She has forgiven me and that She knows that God loves me." He continued, "She says that I must tell Sandy that we are forgiven, because she has been worrying about this also." He seemed to continue the conversation with the image of the Virgin of Guadalupe for several more moments. When it seemed that their conversation was complete, I said gently "Jimmy, none of us know when the hour of our death will arrive, and we don't get to pick exactly what the experience will be like but I have worked with several clients who have found it helpful to consider what their 'ideal death' might be like. Do you have a sense about what your ideal passing might be like?" At first he gave some more intellectually-based comments like "I would not want to be in pain." I then suggested that he reflect on the process of his death. He then took a deep breath and smiled. He said, "I know, when the time of my death comes, the Virgin will appear to me, She will stretch out her arms, and will draw me into them, embracing me as I leave my body." I asked him to ask Her if she was willing to help him in his dying process by attending him as he requested. He smiled as he said with confidence, "Of course She wants to, She has loved me all my life and will even after I die." I then suggested that he might want to spend a few moments rehearsing this part of his death. I asked how he would let Her know that he was ready for Her help. He said that he would raise his arms to Her and She would know it was time. He then spent a few moments practicing this process.

When I asked Jimmy if there was anything else, he said, "No, I am tired" and drifted off to sleep. When I went to see him the next day, the chart reflected that he seemed much less anxious to the hospital staff. He also seemed more relaxed to me. He related that he had liked the imagery session, that he had not thought of the niche in the church for a long time and that he felt better about "his prospects" after death than he had before.

I think in this case Jimmy was able to use imagery to draw on prior positive experiences and have them assist him through the difficult passage of approaching his death. His wife reported that he talked with her more openly about the divorce and remarriage than they ever had and that he was much more comfortable talking about the idea of his death, even though he was not giving up the fight against the cancer. She stated that this was helpful to her even though it was hard because it meant that they could share the pain together.

As a post-script, Jimmy lived about three more weeks after our session. He was able to go home and be with his family and die at home. A hospital bed was set up for Jimmy in the living room and his wife and daughter took turns sitting with him. His daughter reported to me that Jimmy died about one o'clock in the morning. She said he had been sleeping pretty well which had allowed her to doze off. She awoke when he became restless. She tended to him and had just gotten him settled when out of the corner of her eye, she saw him "raise up his arms like a child wanting to be picked up by its mother." She heard him take a single gasping breath and exhale into death with a comforted look upon his face.

On The Other Side of The Bridge

By an imagery practitioner

That morning I felt a wave of emotions as I realized that I was losing one of the very best animal friends I had ever loved. A paralyzing fear engulfed me as I realized just how deep this love went and that Cody, my beautiful sable and white collie, might not be in my life much longer. I had dealt with the loss of other pets before, but Cody was a very special part of my life. There were many times when lying next to him was the only solace I could find.

As I thought about his impending death, I realized that I was at a crossroad – a time for me to make the decision about whether to have him "put to sleep." I knew that I needed to rely on the non-verbal messages from Cody. Being in a relationship with him helped me to develop and trust my intuition, the "unspoken" language. Through intuition, I learned many things about trusting my ability to access the powers of spirituality.

I had attended many a workshop on healing. Certificates for courses on energy work, crystals, yoga, essential oils, meditation, guided imagery and bodywork grace the walls in my office. But, despite all these certificates of learning, on this morning I felt lost. I was faced with not being able to control the outcome and with having to live with the result of my decision. I struggled. I doubted. I suffered. I didn't want to let go.

Six weeks ago I had taken Cody to the vet. It was thought that he was dying and I came close to having him euthanized then, but, just before I signed the papers, Cody awoke. This was a very emotional day for me anyway, because my late brother George's daughter was marrying that very day. I was filled with strong emotions about George not being there for this wonderful day. Cody came out of a near coma, somehow knowing the timing was not right. I considered it his gift to me.

So, here I was once again facing a momentous decision. Part of me was not sure if this was his time. I wanted to make sure that he had every opportunity to recover, but, at the same time, I didn't want him to be in pain or to suffer unnecessarily. From a very deep knowing I thought that we both knew the end was near. Yet, my doubts remained. How did I really know if putting Cody to sleep was the right decision? I hoped against hope that his dying would be his choice, not mine.

In order to reassure myself that I was giving Cody every opportunity to live, I left him at the vet for a series of intravenous infusions. The decision to put him to sleep was put off for a while to see if the IV fluids would produce a change in his condition. It dawned on me that there must be something I could do to find the truth about which choice was best for him, and maybe even for me.

In an attempt to relieve my anxiety about this situation, I tried using my imagery skills to see if the answers truly were within me. I remembered reading an article that explained how imagery was the link to the spiritual world. I have had many vivid and wonderful meditation experiences, but I always wondered if what I experienced was real or just wishful thinking.

Hoping for the best and knowing I would at least relieve some of my tension and anxiety, I relaxed my body and brought forth in my mind an image of my safe place. I imagined a local park where I had spent a great deal of my leisure time with my animals. At the entrance to the park is a large wooden bridge spanning a beautiful rushing stream. As I sat alongside the rushing water I saw, standing on the far side of the bridge, the image of Niki, my dog who I had put to sleep about one year ago. Standing next to Niki was St. Francis of Assisi, patron saint of animals. In the image Niki looked young, vibrant and full of energy. Cody was standing on the near side of the bridge looking fearful and indifferent. I had a sense that

Niki was calling to Cody, telling him it was okay to cross over.

As often happens in the imagery process, I had a sudden inspiration. I remembered how Cody was, in real life, afraid to cross that particular bridge. When Niki was alive and they were together, Cody would always wait until Niki went across first. Then Cody would run across quickly, as if afraid of falling through the planks of the bridge. It seemed that Niki's crossing over first helped Cody have the courage to follow. I was confident that Niki was there to help Cody cross over now.

Coming out of my imagery, I realized that it was time for me to let go and let Cody become whole again – in that great place – wherever that is. I prayed that I would make the right decision for him and realized that he, too, had a choice to live or to die.

I felt confident now that if there was no change in his condition (I was supposed to call the vet at 3 PM), it would be a sign from him that he was choosing spirit over life. I would help him end his suffering—the ultimate selfless act of compassion – letting go. I knew this was a lesson of great proportion for me – a lesson in love, compassion and also of trusting my intuition that the information I received while going within was my truth.

Now, comforted by my imagery experience, I was confident that Cody would be safe and happy being with Niki. I still had hours to go before knowing his condition and making the decision.

Later that day, I found I could no longer stay around the house in anticipation of the call from the vet. I decided to actually drive to the park and write in my journal. Of course, I chose the very same spot that I had seen in my imagery to sit quietly on the bench overlooking the bridge. While there, I set my intention to just let go of Cody and I asked Niki to help him and be with him on his journey. Sensing that I had done all I could do, I got in my car to travel home. I checked the clock – it was 2 PM – only one more hour until I would know Cody's condition and the answer to my dilemma.

As my car approached the bridge, I remembered Cody's fear, closed my eyes and said, "Cody, I'll help you cross this bridge." I felt a great sense of relief as I reached the other side – which was, ironically, marked by a sign saying, "One Way."

When I arrived home, there was a message from my vet asking

me to call right away. The tone in her voice as she answered said it all. And sure enough, Cody's life had come to an end, quietly and peacefully at 2 PM. My tears began to flow and suddenly I remembered in awe that it was the same time I was crossing over the bridge. I had actually helped him cross over that one last time.

The imagery process had guided me toward the right path for both Cody and me. One of the many gifts that Cody gave me is the gift of faith and the gift of experiencing the power of intention. I learned that when I am faced with the painful truths of life and death, I instinctively want to make it better and to take away my pain. When there is nothing else I can do – I can turn to spirit to renew my faith, and to provide comfort and support for myself. I can walk this path we call life – with intention.

Imagery for Health and Wellness

I am certain of nothing but the holiness of the heart's affections and the truth of the imagination.

~ *John Keats*

Healing From Within

By an imagery client

*A*s someone once told me, it only takes one second to change your life forever. My life was changed on April 4, 2003. I was scheduled for spinal reconstruction surgery to correct a spinal curvature. I was told if I chose not to have this surgery I would be permanently looking at the floor in my senior years. Being a registered nurse, the severity of the situation did not escape me. After the surgery, I encountered multiple complications such as three weeks in a coma, bilateral pneumonia and paralysis of my larynx. I was in the Intensive Care Unit for over three months and eventually I was transferred to an Adult Rehabilitation Unit. My physical strength and stamina was at the lowest level that I have ever experienced before in my life. My anxiety level was so high that emotionally I was shell-shocked, trying to grasp the seriousness of my situation and wondering what would be my future, now that my life was changed forever.

I knew if I were ever going to achieve the highest level of healing that I would need to incorporate all modalities of healing. It is my belief that utilizing both traditional medicine and alternative healing practices is essential to achieve optimal health. I was extremely fortunate that the hospital offered various complementary healing techniques such as healing massage, body energy work and creative imagery.

My first encounter with imagery was to create an imaginary sanctuary where I could meet my inner healers. My special place is a beautiful green meadow, with a tall oak tree and a running clear brook. My healers introduced themselves to me with such love and compassion that I knew they were my partners in this healing journey. Each session, I was guided by a certified Integrative Imagery professional, who gently encouraged my own healing process.

I was told by the physician that I may have to do self-catheterizations due to my inability to urinate following the effects of the spinal surgery on my bladder. In the imagery session, one of my inner healers named Jessica came to assist me in working with my bladder. When the time came for me to either void or be catheterized, I began to imagine Jessica's hands over my bladder. This felt as if energy was being sent to the areas where it was needed and I began to void on my own. I no longer had to do the self-catheterizations. I knew that I could continue to call upon Jessica. She has proven to be faithful and highly competent in her assigned duty to assist me.

This experience was so huge for me that I actually felt I was no longer alone in this process of recovery. I have an inner world of healers that are loving and available to me as I travel on this path of healing. I believe that these inner healers are aspects of my own inner wisdom and have my best and loving interest in mind at all times. It could be described as connecting to the Divine source where the inner healing can be accessed. It is truly becoming a participant in one's own healing. In times of crisis and feelings of defeat it allows one to feel empowered and capable of helping oneself to heal.

As I continued on this journey, I was eventually diagnosed with osteomyelitis (an infection in the bone) of the lumbar spine. I was devastated and the pain was so intense that I finally lost hope that I was ever going to be able to heal. My feelings were so overwhelming that I began supportive psychotherapy during a prolonged hospitalization period. I was able to recall my sessions with my imagery guide, and continued to go within to my sanctuary to feel safe. The imagery guide kept in touch by phone and sent me healing tapes to do in preparation for further surgeries. As I look back at this time, I do not believe I would have gotten through so many set backs if I did not have this new resource of creative imagery and inner healing.

I eventually returned to my home where, after being in bed for four months because of the osteomyelitis, I had developed osteoporosis (loss of normal bone density). As I was walking, I crushed my right knee severely. I returned to the hospital yet again. Working with my imagery guide and my inner healers, I developed a plan to combat the osteoporosis. Two new inner healers appeared in my imagery. Tony and Sheila were in charge of "painting" all my bones with a specialized white formula that was blessed at the inner holy altar in my sanctuary. This formula assisted the new bone cells to form and I visualized Tony and Sheila's painting daily. When the time came for the total knee replacement, the orthopedic specialist remarked how much bone there was to work with, something he never thought would have occurred in this length of time. A total knee replacement was successfully completed August 22, 2005.

I have had many occasions to work with my inner healing guides. Jonathan was the one who assisted me in controlling persistent diarrhea from the multiple courses of antibiotics. He helps me with another formula specifically designed to strengthen the immune system. To this day, he continues to work with me since this has been an ongoing need for my healing.

During a difficult time of feeling defeated and having to deal with such intense pain, I met again with my imagery guide to do a session to address all of these difficult feelings. I knew that I was into old feelings and dealing with multiple bladder infections was very frightening. We went to my special place in the meadow to connect with my healing inner guides. They were quite conscious of the emotional state I was in and they came as a group with a very soft gentle blue baby blanket and wrapped it all around me. I felt the softness and the caring of these inner healers and they knew that I just needed to be loved. They weren't there to change the feelings or to come up with solutions. They were just there to allow me to feel loved. I felt the genuineness of this love and it immediately allowed me to feel calm and remember that I am always loved. I was able to cope, not in a state of emotional upheaval, but in a state of calm and love to effectively deal with many issues confronting me. And now whenever I need to, I wrap myself in the blue blanket of love.

The creative imagery process has been such a dynamic tool for self-healing over three years now. I have developed a loving, caring attitude towards myself and an awareness of my body that I never had before. I lived my life not being aware that I had a body until it finally presented itself with so much pain I knew I had to become sensitive to its needs. Awareness, development of a healing sanctuary and the loving relationships of my healers continue to help me live a life of consciousness. Even though I am now disabled, I am living a life full of love and actively staying in the present moment. This divine presence is where one can find love, harmony and joy. And through these, the body can accomplish amazing feats. I have now returned to working part time and I am even able to cope with the challenges of travel. I am also proud to say I am healthy enough to be in the training program to learn to be an Integrative Imagery guide.

The Power of Example

By a student guide

*D*on is an Emergency Room physician who worked with me, a registered nurse studying Integrative Imagery. I had been using the imagery in the emergency department to help patients with anxiety and painful situations. Don and the rest of the staff would overhear me talking with patients while starting their IVs or giving medications to help them relax. "Just take some slow deep breaths, Mr. 'Smith,' and let your body's natural pain relief, the endorphins, release to help the pain subside and the muscles relax. Picture yourself on that beach you were telling me about and feel the warm sun on your back while you rest on the sand."

The staff did not necessarily believe any of this talking would really impact the patient's physical status but it often did help the patients to calm down a bit and that usually helps everyone in a busy and stressful place. Don and a few of the other doctors began to appreciate it more when doing procedures that required moderate anesthesia. Often patients needed to have dislocated joints reduced into place or wound cleaning and repair that required extra pain management and sedation. During those times I would talk with the patient before the procedure to explain what to expect and answer any questions. Also, I would inquire if the person had a special place to go when celebrating, taking time out from life, or feeling low and needing to re-group. With the person's permission, while giving the medications, I would talk with them during the procedure to assist them to imagine being in that special place. The patients would report that they enjoyed that personal support and they felt the procedure was not as bad as they thought it might be. Often the patients did not require quite as much sedation from the medications, which shortens their recovery time. The physicians are satisfied when the patient is safe, co-operative, well managed for comfort and the procedure usually goes well.

One day Don was on duty and needed to take care of a patient with an infected wound. The patient was a middle-aged man named "Joe." Joe was quite agitated and while he wanted the medical care, he could not assure Dr. Don that he would be able to stay quiet and still while the doctor injected the local anesthetic, cleaned, and packed the wound. Don offered Joe the option of some extra medications to help him relax. The nurse on duty started the IV and gave the medications as ordered. They began the procedure giving more medications when necessary. The patient was trying to be still but was becoming a bit "squirrelly" in Don's words. They had already given quite a bit of medication to this patient. Don thought to himself, 'what would our imagery nurse say if she were here to help this guy settle down?' So, he said to the patient, "Joe, listen for a minute. Now just try to relax and tell me if you could be anywhere in the world right now, where would you be?" The patient appeared to relax his body a bit and stop to think. Then he got a big grin on his face and replied, "Oh hell, Doc, that's easy. I'd be at the Sunrise Bunny Ranch outside of Reno!" "Well Joe, I really don't need to hear any more about that. You just enjoy thinking about all that and I'll be done here in just a few minutes." The patient stayed quiet while Don quickly finished the procedure.

Even though Don and many of the other physicians and nurses have thought this was just a lot of "spiritual or mental mumbo-jumbo and fluff" they noticed it was effective. And Don was willing to try it. The power of example is strong.

Dr. Don learned it was easy to do imagery but was also surprised with Joe's words and was not sure how to respond at first. I guess education and training for this is important.

I think Don did well and am so happy he found a way to help "Joe" and himself get through the procedure.

For me the lesson was: Don't be shy about doing what you know can help people!

Messages from Jesus

By a student guide

As someone who is a light sleeper, I could identify easily with my sixty-three-year-old patient. Her arthritis, both in her left shoulder and in her left hip often caused her to wake up because of the pain and because she was such a light sleeper. She asked for help, saying she would like to be able to fall asleep easily (sometimes she is awake for hours before actually falling asleep) and stay asleep every night.

Marian was very familiar and comfortable with the imagery process that she learned from her therapist. I did a very detailed head-to-toe relaxation with Marian, focusing on breathing and suggesting that she "take in what you need and let go of what you don't need." After about ten minutes of this process Marian nodded her head as a signal that she was ready to begin the imagery work. Marian's special place was a beautiful garden with many bright flowers, a small pond with a fountain in the center. There was a large tree with grassy area and an inviting bench underneath the tree. Marian imagined herself sitting on the bench under the tree, but she still had the feeling something was missing. When I asked her what she felt was missing from this picture, she realized that there were no animals or birds singing. After a moment of reflection, she said there was a puppy near her snuggling up close.

We then invited an inner healer figure to come forward. Marian said the healer within her was God and Jesus came forward to help her, sitting comfortably next to her on the bench underneath the tree. As she looked at Him, she noticed especially, His large, strong, kind hands. He was very gentle and had hands that could heal anything with His touch. He was wearing a white robe and had very large shoulders (the kind that could support you always).

When Marian asked Jesus what she needed to help her sleep at night, she was surprised that Jesus mentioned that she usually asked for things for other people, rather than for herself. He told her He would always be there and to trust in Him and that He would always love and support her. He also encouraged her to pray to Him and to believe that He would help her take away all the other thoughts that keep her awake. He reminded her that when she took the time to ask for something for herself, He would be quick to comply. He told her she was learning to be more comfortable with asking for things for herself. She thanked the Jesus figure for coming and agreed that in the future she would pray for what she needed.

As nurturers, women often put others before themselves. This woman learned, in a very powerful way, from a very powerful inner wisdom figure, that it was OK to ask for help for herself in a self-caring, gentle and loving way.

Things Are Not Always What They Appear to Be

By a student guide

*I*ntegrative Imagery has been a powerful and amazing tool for me. It has allowed me to connect with my inner self on many levels, providing answers and guiding my direction. The power of this process was evidenced in the very first session that I guided a fellow student through the exercise of imagining yourself in a special place. This experience occurred on our second day of imagery class, as I held the recommended script in my hand. My "client" was a nurse, working full time in a hospital. She wanted to find a special place to relax to help with the pain she gets frequently from migraine headaches. The frequency and intensity of the headaches was increasing over the last year. Her medical workup included CT scans, an MRI and full physicals, yet no source could be found for the continuing headaches. They were precipitated and became worse under stress, especially long stretches at work. Medication provided some relief for her, but she didn't want to depend on meds. She was single and lived alone. She agreed to try the imagery to find a special place to relax.

After guiding her through progressive relaxation, she formed an image of her special place. She was on a beach; the air was warm, with a gentle breeze. The sky was blue with a few sea gulls flying by and she could smell the salty ocean air. She was sitting on the warm sand, gazing out over the ocean listening to the gentle breaking of the waves on the seashore which formed a nice rhythm. As she looked out on the horizon, she saw a huge sailboat gently sailing into view. The boat was far away but coming closer, sailing parallel to the shore. She was just sitting, watching the boat sail by. As it came into view, she noticed the sails were black. The next thing I knew she was crying. I asked her if she was OK and she replied yes. I asked her what was happening and she said the boat was talking to her. I asked her if she wanted to stop but she said she wanted to know what the boat was doing in her special place. I told her to ask. She did that and then the tears really flowed. The boat told her "It's OK to quit your job."

When I asked if she was alright she responded yes. She didn't want to stop yet. She said the boat told her it was ok to quit her job. It had no other messages for her. When she was ready, she thanked the boat and said goodbye and it faded away. She then rested in her special place for a short while. As she let the image of her special place fade, and opened her eyes, she was crying.

This whole experience was making no sense to me. I thought relaxing in a special place would make someone feel happy. I didn't expect it to be so emotional, nor did I expect her reflection on the process. She stated that she had worked at her job for twenty years, and her father had been a nurse at the same hospital until he retired. He always mentioned what a wonderful job it was, and how his benefits and pension were so good. He would say, "Stay here until you retire. It's the best job around for security and pension."

She started to cry saying that as the black sail boat was speaking to her, she was hearing her father's voice in her mind, even though he had died a number of years ago. She had forgotten that he had given that advice about job security at the hospital. Apparently over the last year she had gone on a couple of job interviews in an attempt to change jobs, but just couldn't make the decision to do it, and she didn't know why. One of the offers was good and she didn't know what held her back. Now it all made sense to her. She thanked me and I didn't see her until four months later at our next phase of imagery training.

I didn't recognize her when she ran up to me and gave me a hug. Her hair was cut short; she lost about 15 pounds, she had quit her job, and loved her new job, and had not experienced a migraine since the imagery session. I was really amazed; in fact both of us were. This was my first dramatic, life changing experience with Integrative Imagery. I felt it was a true justification of the power of the process and not the experience of the guide, as it had been my first time guiding. Throughout that first session I kept feeling confused-this black ship made no sense to me-I needed to trust in the process. By trusting in the process and allowing this to be "her" experience she was able to bring all this information out of her subconscious and deal with it. The emotional release was frightening for both of us. Remembering this, I always caution clients that they may experience an emotional release during an imagery session. It was important to note that her migraines were worked up from a medical standpoint because headaches can be a sign of severe medical conditions.

Looking back I see this sailboat as a symbol of moving on, as a symbol of freedom. From a traditional Chinese medicine standpoint, the color black is related to the Kidney (acupuncture) channel, water and the emotion of fear. That would explain the black ship, floating on the water and that "thing" that held her back from accepting "good" job offers. However, this was her experience not mine. But I can tell you that I will never see a solitary sailboat floating across the ocean without thinking of her and realizing the tremendous power that we possess to help ourselves heal. Being a guide in this sacred journey is both a joy and a privilege.

A Moment in Time

By an imagery guide

*W*ithin my private practice, I have been honored to be witness to many magical moments in which an individual makes the decision to use imagery as a tool, discovering the beauty and power of their own personal wisdom. It is truly amazing that when Integrative Imagery is experienced, it is as if a hidden pathway has been uncovered, allowing the individual to access a deeper level of understanding when needed, even if least expected or planned. When I first met Martha she had already seen a wide variety of health care professionals, both conventional and alternative, for longstanding, persistent physical symptoms. She had undergone years of repeated tests, investigations and consultations but found no relief from her distress. Her daily life and the majority of her conversation revolved around her symptom experiences. It had become all consuming and friends had started to drift away. Martha and I spoke about the relaxation response, the mind-body connection and the process of Integrative Imagery. I invited her to consider the possibility of using imagery as a self-help tool. She had exhausted most other routes and was eager to give it a try.

Our first imagery session went very well. Martha, a well-educated, older woman, was very gifted in the arts and she easily accessed images as she explored her special place. She described in detail the splash of colorful flowers nestled by foliage, heard the call of early birds at the brink of dawn, and smiled as she described the feeling of cool morning dew on her feet. Her face lit up with delight as she drew in the fresh smells of a new day, experienced the feeling of being flooded with energy by the rays of the rising sun and tasted the sweet tang of lemonade as the heat of the sun exploded into hot summer air. Martha looked and felt relaxed and rejuvenated at the end of the session. During our second session, Martha said that she had decided that she wanted to use a tool more specific to her symptoms. We agreed to work on an imagery scale of 10 (most intense) to 1 (least intense or pain-free) to help reduce the intensity of her pain and symptom experience. Again, Martha accessed images easily as Integrative Imagery allowed her intensity scale to be tailored to her life experiences by changing the usual 10 to 1 scale to a written musical scale complete with the sound of the notes and colors. Following the imagery, Martha said she felt less anxious and less distressed by her symptoms. It appeared that all had gone well in introducing Martha to two potentially powerful imagery tools.

I was surprised, when during our third session, she flatly refused to use imagery anymore. She had not used either of the imagery techniques between visits. Her symptoms had escalated and her mind focused on her symptom pattern. Together we had talked about the mind-body connection, a familiar topic to Martha, and the benefits of the relaxation response. Martha had easily accessed and worked with the images in both sessions and seemed pleased with the resultant experiences. It had appeared to be such a natural fit. What had suddenly changed? Martha's explanation was simple. Her symptoms were not in her head so she wasn't going to work with her mind. Martha had made her decision and was adamant that imagery was not for her. She made it very clear that she was not open to any discussion on the matter or to her feelings surrounding her decision.

Over the course of the next few months, we worked together using other tools. We focused on facilitating the relaxation response, supporting the continuous growth of the nurse-client relationship and finding ways to create for Martha moments of respite from her continuous symptoms. One early spring day during a session Martha, who was housebound, asked me a question about the effects of the heavy spring rains that we had just had in the area. I described the scene in my own front yard and accompanied the description with some "squishy mud" sound effects. As Martha heard the sounds, the look on her face suddenly changed. It changed so much that I immediately stopped. She looked far off into the distance and started to reminisce by spontaneously launching into a description of a memory from her youth, vividly full of wonderful sensory images---sights, sounds, smells, tastes, textures and the emotions associated with the memory. At that moment and for the next 20 minutes, Martha was transported to that time so long ago. With her eyes wide open, no defined imagery session planned and no specific relaxation preparation, Martha excitedly explored this meaningful image from her past. With little more than a quick confirmation that she was comfortable sharing this moment and "holding the space," the process unfolded in an amazing and beautiful way. I knew that, both intuitively and from the content of our conversations over the previous few months, Martha had graced me with her permission to share this special moment and she willingly engaged in the imagery process again in my presence. As her image began to fade and she started to withdraw from the active imagery process, her eyes welled with tears and her face softened from joyful, excitement to tender gratitude. She smiled and whispered, "I feel so peaceful. Thank you for this-it has meant more to me than you could ever know."

Martha still did not participate in any specific imagery sessions. At times, if she felt comfortably open, we would talk about imagery. I would invite her to use images and then we would discuss her imagery process together. At other times there was again a strong resistance on her part to anything that involved looking inward. It seemed, however, from that point on Martha found more and more comfort and peace in her life. Her daily activities became less focused on her symptoms and she rediscovered her sharp sense of humor. Slowly, Martha began to take interest in the relationships in her life again.

Five years later, I saw Martha again as she neared the end of her life journey. She eagerly shared with me images related to her spirituality and the meaningful messages that she received through these powerful and meaningful images.

I have learned that sometimes, for whatever reason, I have been given the opportunity to introduce imagery to someone and to just simply open the door of possibility. Just opening the door can be enough, and as the guide I must trust the body's innate wisdom of how and when to best use this wonderful tool. The potential un-folding of an imagery process often seems to lie waiting for just the right moment in time to exquisitely rise to the surface, bringing with it incredible transformative power and beauty.

Imagery for Cancer and Treatment

I am imagination. I can see what the eyes cannot see. I can hear what the ears cannot hear. I can feel what the heart cannot feel.

~ Peter Nivio Zarlenga

The Owl and the Eagle

By an imagery client

*I*n July of 1999, I was diagnosed with ovarian cancer, stage IV. I had a hysterectomy and the removal of a very large tumor. Following surgery I began chemotherapy. The standard treatment for ovarian cancer is Taxol and Carboplatin, but the first day of chemotherapy I had an anaphylactic (severe allergic) reaction to the Taxol. It was very severe, and I was told I couldn't take the drug again. However, my doctor wanted to make sure, so he introduced it again 3 weeks later, in the hospital. I immediately reacted, so the chemotherapy drugs were changed to Carboplatin and Cytoxin. I finally completed treatment in January of 2000. Sadly, 6 months later the tumor marker numbers began to rise and my oncologist said it was time to do chemotherapy again, and that he wanted to try the Taxol one more time.

I was terribly depressed about the recurrence and frightened about having another cycle of chemotherapy treatments. I was having a lot of trouble handling the emotional stress of the situation and decided that I could either take sedatives or try something different. I began guided imagery a few weeks before the chemotherapy was scheduled to begin. The imagery was natural and easy for me and during my first session I found myself in my childhood bedroom, resting on my bed. It was wonderful to feel so safe. I expected to have my deceased grandmother enter through the door, but instead a huge owl appeared at the window. In my imagination, we began to talk about my disease and the treatment.

On the day of treatment, the doctor decided to try the Taxol again. I was surrounded by nurses, my oncologist and the pharmacist. They acted calm, but we all knew it was because they needed to be prepared for another emergency. The IV drip began and nothing happened. I didn't have a reaction. My doctor attributed it to his skill and luck, but I had a different idea. I believed that it was the guided imagery because for several days before the treatment I'd been working with my owl and a personalized guided imagery tape. During the imagery process, the owl and I had been joined by an eagle and we made a plan for the day of treatment. The owl would take my place and receive the Taxol, because he was used to the active ingredient, which comes from the yew tree. He said it wouldn't affect him. The eagle agreed that he would take me away on his back during treatment so I wouldn't need to be present at all. It was no surprise to me that on the day of treatment all went according to plan, and I was able to tolerate the drug.

Over the course of the cancer and treatments, many "inner allies" have appeared in my imagery. The following is a list of the "guides" that joined me the first year, and the qualities that I associate with them:

Owl – wisdom, intelligence, good counsel, patience

Eagle – courage and strength

Ferret – (three ferrets) ability to search in hidden places to ferret out the cancer cells

Rabbit – he became the main advisor, choosing the right diet, intuition, leadership, persistence

Old Stag – advice and the wisdom that comes with age. He has spent years avoiding death

American Indian maiden and warrior brave – represented feminine and masculine spiritual guidance, warrior qualities to fight the disease

Wolf/Dog – playfulness, spirit of youth

Bear- helped when the cancer in the spine caused a great deal of leg pain

A few other guides joined for one or two sessions. Among them was Dr. Fox, who bore a striking resemblance to my oncologist. Also, there was an ethereal spirit-being who gave me spiritual guidance. My grandmother was also a part of the imagery, but she "lived" in another spot in a garden I created that was located in the bowl of my pelvis. She had made a beautiful sunny spot filled with flowers and she was always there sending me love and comfort.

The Taxol wasn't as successful as we'd hoped, and the tumor marker numbers began to rise again. This time I was given Doxil, another type of chemotherapy. Again, I worked with my guides to manage the drug. I was able to take the Doxil for three years, which I've been told is quite unusual. I had only minor reactions to the drug, and while on it I took a trip to Italy and also began horseback riding lessons and Italian classes, as well as returning to work.

The Doxil had a side effect of mouth sores, and in September of 2003 one of them suddenly turned into a squamous cell cancer on my upper palate. I turned to my guides for help. The rabbit played a leadership role, and the others stationed themselves inside my mouth to keep the cancer contained. I had surgery to remove the cancer with remarkably little pain. The guides worked with my immune system to help me heal. Doxil was discontinued. The oral cancer has not returned.

In June of 2004 I had another recurrence of ovarian cancer, a tumor near one kidney and tumors on my lower spine. I was given Taxol and Carboplatin again. The tumors shrank. In March of 2005 my tumor marker numbers again began to rise, so I began a regimen of Chinese herbs and other supplements. I also worked with guided imagery to help control the cancer and also to help the supplements work more effectively.

Just after beginning the new regimen I had an important dream. I woke up with my heart beating hard and feeling very frightened. In the dream I saw that I'd been letting a panther live in my house, even though it had been hurting me and scaring me. A few days later I had a session of guided imagery, and in it one of my original guides, the playful wolf/dog, turned into a massive Irish wolfhound and nipped the heels of the panther as it was loaded into a crate for transport to the Brazilian rain forest. The Wolf remains on guard at the door of my house to keep the panther away. In subsequent work with the tape, a large black bear guide has joined the dog to patrol the perimeter of my home. Once I realized the panther was a bully, I became proactive to go after it. When I did, it became small, meek and harmless.

Imagery has become a seamless part of my life. For instance, while receiving acupuncture, I looked into my body and saw the stag wanting to communicate with me. The acupuncturist had been working with my kidneys for a number of sessions, and the stag was there to help with the kidneys, too. The image that I saw was the stag walking on my kidneys with his small pointed hooves, helping to stimulate them, similar to the needles of acupuncture. Another time, during radiation, I looked into my body and saw several of the guides wearing protective clothing and eyewear, holding back sensitive skin so that the radiation would go straight to the spine where the cancer was located. Any time I look into my body I can immediately connect with the guides and see what they are doing. I most often do this when I am meditating or having a treatment.

Sometimes I ask the guides for specific advice, such as how to handle a side effect or an emotion. An especially helpful piece of advice was that I flow with the cancer rather than fight it. At first I rebelled at the idea, but later realized it was exactly what I'd been doing all along, considering the complementary therapies I'd been using. I also ask the guides for protection from the side effects of radiation or chemotherapy. They always respond right away by going to the sensitive site in my body with whatever protection was necessary. During radiation they put protective blankets around my organs, and during chemotherapy they wrapped my healthy cells in a heavy plastic coating until the drug had dissipated.

The most vivid and interesting images come to me during guided imagery sessions. In the days that follow a session I find that the images evolve and change to give me more benefit. When my deceased grandmother first appeared in a garden in my pelvis during a session, I was thrilled. Each day when I visited her, the garden had gotten more elaborate and covered a larger portion of my pelvis, giving me more protection. When my mother died, an image of her joined my grandmother in the garden and I am able to visit them and get advice and strength from them whenever I need.

This story doesn't do full justice to the spiritual journey I've been on for all these years. I feel that my work with guided imagery has been a huge part of why I'm still alive and healthy. The work has helped me calm my fears and face the possibility of death, which has been very empowering. Every time I've needed advice or help, my guides have come forward with an answer. I've found a spiritual side of myself, as well as discovered that my intuition is a wonderful gift. These two qualities have added richness to my life in more ways then I could have imagined.

Post note by Joan's imagery practitioner
Joan died Monday, November 20, 2006.

Joan once referred to herself as the poster child for complementary therapy. Oh no, she is so much more. She is a miracle, having lived seven and a half years with stage IV ovarian cancer and active disease a large portion of that time. The chemotherapy, no doubt, kept the cancer at bay. But it was her indomitable spirit and her successful use of her magical imagery, Chinese medicine and energy therapies that enabled her to live well for that span of time.

During the last two months of her life Joan did not want to do any active imagery. I trust, though, that her animal allies and her ancestors were all close by through her tedious decline. Her magical inner world reflected her ingenious, creative life-loving spirit. She lived her life well and sadly died all too soon. And all along the way, she graced so many of us with her beautiful spirit.

Joan, may you fly free with your owl and your eagle.

Carolyn's Angel

By an imagery guide

*C*arolyn gingerly lowered herself into the chair until her head, neck, and shoulders were fully supported under the smooth, rounded form of the cushions. Once settled into their soft contours, she carefully placed her aching legs on the ottoman in front of her. It had been two months since she learned her breast cancer had returned and metastasized into her bones. Her inner struggle to remain hopeful and stay strong was beginning to feel like a losing battle. "Will this imagery really help?" she wondered aloud.

She gently closed her eyes and began to take deep, slow breaths. It seemed that with each exhalation she surrendered more and more into the comfort and relaxation that was beginning to envelop her. The tension and pain that had held such a severe grip on her body was at last releasing and melting away. Feeling completely suspended in time, and in this wonderful state of tranquility, her thoughts began to transport her to a serene and magnificent healing place. She began to speak.

"There is a waterfall, and while the air is cool, the sand is very warm beneath my feet, and it feels so good. It is just so beautiful and peaceful here. I would like to find a comfortable place in the warm sand and stay a while." Sighing deeply, she tilted her head slightly, and continued her train of thought.

"Close beside me where I am sitting on the sand there is a rock with brilliant white lights emanating from it. It is amazing as one of the lights is sparkling like a diamond and somehow I know these lights have been waiting for me. How strange though-as the lights don't really have any form-they are just beautiful lights, and yet I have this sense that they are here for a reason. I feel like they have

something to tell me."

It wasn't long before soft tears began to roll gently down her cheeks. "The light that is sparkling like a diamond is beginning to transform itself. I can't believe what is happening. It is just all so surreal. It is my beloved dog Tasha, who died eight years ago. She is walking out of the diamond of light toward me with her tender eyes of understanding looking into my soul."

Even through closed eyes, it appeared as though Carolyn were looking directly into the very gaze that she was describing. "I, I can't stop crying," she said. "I believe God has sent her as an Angel to be here with me again."

"Tasha stood by me and brought me so much love and comfort during my chemotherapy treatments with my breast cancer ten years ago. I want her to stay and help ease my pain. She is giving me kisses, and is laying her head on my sore rib. She is telling me she has come to bring me comfort and relieve my pain during this difficult time, and she will help me find the inner strength to deal with what lies before me. These tears are tears of joy because I feel so comforted. My heart is overflowing with gratitude right now."

"I know I will remember this sense of well being in my body for as long as I live by simply placing my hands over my heart. It will bring me back to this special healing place and Tasha's loving, big, black eyes telling me she will not leave my side. All I need to do is call for her."

Carolyn suddenly became very quiet as she rested in the love and compassion that she felt all around her. The reunion with her late companion moved her and touched her so deeply that she did not want to leave. But as the tears dried, she said good-bye and reluctantly reopened her eyes. They clearly reflected a renewed sense of hope.

It wasn't long after this session took place with my sister that she required surgery on a tumor that was growing near her clavicle. When I asked her if she wanted me to be there for the early morning procedure she said it wasn't necessary, and that our mother would be with her. But I wasn't totally convinced it was the right thing not to go, so I prayed the night before her surgery. My prayer went something like this: "God if you want me to show up for this surgery and it is important that I be there please help me wake up early in the morning."

I went to sleep, but at about 5:30 AM I woke up to the loud sound of a barking dog. I could have sworn the dog was in the house and right outside my bedroom door, but how could it possibly be? My dog was snoozing away in her dog bed without a sound. I listened quietly and heard it again. My dog was still snoozing away, yet the bark seemed to be so near the room. It was then I realized this was the wake-up call to be present at the hospital. When I walked into the waiting room, I could feel Carolyn's gratitude. I had made the right decision.

I shared this story with Carolyn before she went into surgery, and we had a good laugh together as I told her how much I appreciated the visit from her "Angel." This was very reassuring for both of us to actually see how her faith and imagery were already supporting her in such a tangible way.

It has been more than two years since my sister and I held this imagery session together. Not only has it brought us closer, but I will always be grateful for the rich experience and the great lesson it taught me about the power of being fully present in every moment. When called upon, Tasha still comes and brings my sister gentle comfort. And it is through that gentle comfort that imagery has continued to be a powerful tool which supports, inspires, helps heal, and gives great insight into all aspects of our lives.

A New View of Chemotherapy

By an imagery guide

*H*aving recently had a lumpectomy for breast cancer, Carla came to see me because she was going to begin a course of chemotherapy in about two weeks. She was feeling very nervous about the chemo (particularly the side effects) and wanted to create images that might help her get over her fear and be able to "view" the chemo in a more positive light. As we talked, Carla shared that she felt "up and down" about her ability to cope with her diagnosis. "It's like I'm getting it in layers. Some days I'm feeling really strong and positive and sometimes I wake up in the middle of the night feeling terrified. I do feel, though, like I'm coming to grips with my diagnosis a little better each day."

She had used a pre-operative guided imagery CD before her lumpectomy and had found it very helpful in helping her stay relaxed before the procedure, but she was new to Integrative Imagery. I explained the process to her and we began our session with a slow and leisurely progressive relaxation. During the process I was acutely aware of my own feelings of empathy toward her and my desire to help her create a space where she could feel relaxed and safe. When she indicated she was ready to proceed, I invited her to imagine that she was receiving her first dose of chemo and was watching it work inside her body. She was quite still for a bit and then laughed softly. "It's like a flock of miniature angels— white and 'shimmery' with magic horns. They aim the horns at the cancer cells and blow them away. They just turn to dust."

I asked, "The cancer cells turn to dust?"

"Yes," she said, "and they make a funny crunching sound, sort of like taking a handful of potato chips and squeezing hard." She laughed softly again.

I asked her a few more questions and Carla described the way the angels moved. "They don't sweep like I'd expect – they're more like pin-balls, pinging around and looking for cancer cells. They're very fast and somehow …joyful…and competent. They know just what they're doing."

After a few more minutes, I asked Carla to check in with her body and to describe how these angels were making her body feel.

"It's humming…very vibrant…there's a lot going on. It's important and….just very active, vital and smart." I invited her to enjoy the feeling of vibrancy and activity. She was quiet for quite a while then offered, "I feel very light --filled with light. Light but strong, like I'm not going to be blown off-course by this. I can do this."

After allowing her time to stay with the feeling of lightness, I encouraged her to hold the memory of the angels and the feeling of vibrant light and then to slowly let the images fade. I allowed her time to come back into her body and to more conscious awareness.

In talking with Carla after the session, she expressed surprise and amusement in the images that came to her during her session. "They're my own little flock of avenging angels!" She commented that she really appreciated the relaxation phase and felt very loved and protected as she transitioned to the imaginal state. She also stated that she felt much less nervous about the upcoming chemo treatments now that she knew she could invite in a flock of angels to blast the cancer cells with their trumpets. She appeared relaxed and energized – much calmer and grounded than she seemed before the imagery session.

Wisdom for Making a Difficult Decision

By an imagery guide

*K*elley was a thirty-eight-year-old married woman with four young children who had been diagnosed with stage III breast cancer. She had sought out my services as a healing coach many months before and participated in a series of healing touch sessions with me. She received chemotherapy 20 times. Out of our coaching sessions, she decided to see a naturopath and started taking many herbs and supplements. She had many healing classes and sessions with a Qigong master. She visited a faith healer from her church and sought council from many who had been through the cancer experience already. She had a strong Christian faith.

Now she was scheduled for a bilateral mastectomy this week. She asked if she could try guided imagery because she was making what she thought was the most important decision of her life. After all of this treatment, her PET scan showed no evidence of cancer. With this information she went back to her Qigong master who said he saw no cancer anywhere. The faith healer independently said he saw no cancer anywhere and that there were only two times when he had seen people where he felt there was an instant healing and that she had been one of those. Her oncologist and the surgeon both recommended the surgery saying that the PET scan could not pick up the microscopic evidence of cancer and there was no guarantee it was gone. Her family and friends were all expecting her to have the surgery, but she had put it on hold.

Kelley said she had made an appointment with me to help her get some clarity on all of this and possibly do guided imagery. She arrived utterly at odds about whether or not to have the surgery. She was in a dilemma, saying that after God had delivered so much healing, she worried that if she decided to have the surgery God might be upset with her for not having enough faith. She was concerned that He might withdraw His support from her.

That's when I suggested that we have a talk about God. We ended up clarifying her beliefs in her God, talking about unconditional love, about all the tools He gave her and that one of those tools might be surgery. She also mentioned that she has always had to have two opinions on things to feel it was right.

That settled, we discussed what her session would be that evening, and she decided she wanted to find an inner wisdom figure. I took her through a head to toe relaxation and asked her to go to a place of safety and comfort. She went to her bedroom in her mother's house. She described the bedroom in detail. She was standing looking out the window into the woods. I asked her to invite someone who loved her very much and knew her well to come to her. She said there were two figures in the woods, one a deer and one an eagle. I was quite sure the wisdom figure was the eagle, but I asked her to ask the one which was there as her wisdom figure that evening to step forth. When I asked what was happening, Kelley said she was holding the eagle in her arms. It felt really light and she went on to describe its yellow beak and dark eyes. "What I really notice is its head. It's looking at me like it knows."

When asked why it came, she said it felt to her as if it wanted to show her something. "The eagle wants me to fly somewhere with it." I told her to climb on and go. Now she was soaring above the woods and above the lake. "He is showing me that I am strong, like him." I asked what that was like for her and she said, "I feel so free. It's freedom."

I instructed her to stay with the eagle and absorb this feeling of freedom, giving her lots of time. There were tears. (As the guide I recognized that it had to be remarkable for her to be away from the concerns and worries of cancer in her life.) Then I told her to ask eagle about the surgery. He nodded his head. I asked what that meant to her and she said it meant it was the right thing to go ahead with the surgery. I asked how she was with that and she said she felt serious. Kelley's image changed and she was in the operating room now. Her Grandma was there smiling and watching. Kelley was feeling afraid and I told her to ask for the eagle and he came immediately. He was sitting on her chest, but she was still feeling scared. I instructed her to tell that to eagle and he then was flying her up toward the mountains where it was green.

When I asked her what this image meant to her she said that her Grandma symbolizes peace and understanding. She has been in my place before. She wanted me to know what she learned, that you have to use the doctors. She didn't, and then it was too late for her.

When I asked Kelley if there was anything else she said she wanted the eagle to stay, but he couldn't because he had to fly free. I then asked her how she could get in contact with him if she felt she needed him. "I just have to reach out and he'll fly back into my arms."

At the end of the session, I asked her how she was and she said, "peaceful." It was clear to me that this woman had not experienced peacefulness since her diagnosis. She said she was better. "I don't have to do it alone. Someone else can show me the way. I'm tired of figuring it out. Someone else can be in charge." She also talked about the feeling of flying free again.

We took a moment to confirm that she felt surgery was the right decision. She was at peace with it and definitely knew she would do it. She said that it felt good to know that and she knew she wouldn't waver. I also mentioned to her that she had said earlier that she needs two opinions to feel something is right and that perhaps her grandmother came to confirm the eagle's "yes" answer to surgery. She was very excited about that.

My Guides

By an imagery client

$\mathcal{I}$ became enchanted with the power of imagery after I was diagnosed with cancer of the parotid gland in 1996. As my world came crashing down around me, I scrambled to find some therapies that would help me deal with my fears. Not only was I concerned about the cancer itself, I was also concerned about the physical symptoms that were occurring due to the treatments. After undergoing surgery for removal of the parotid gland and lymph nodes I began 6 weeks of radiation therapy to the head and neck area. Using imagery throughout the entire process and for several years after proved to be a profound experience for me. It was transformative in many ways, a few of which I elucidate here.

My first use of imagery was to help me get through the radiation treatments without being frightened every time I went to the hospital. I was very afraid of what radiation would do to me. It had partially caused my illness because I had radiation to my adenoids when I was only five year's old. Ironically, the radiation that would supposedly "cure" me had caused the problem in the first place!

In the imagery I addressed my concerns about the radiation treatments. I visualized a grotto and an underground crystal cave where dolphins were swimming in the ocean for my pleasure and joy. Every day of my treatment I would see the sun shining into my crystal cave and the radiation rays would beam off of the crystals and transform the rays into healing rays directed at my neck. To minimize the effects of the radiation, I would imagine diving into the ocean and swimming with my beautiful dolphins. Rather than being frightened during the treatments, I found when I did my positive visualization, it made me feel so much better about what I was doing and my fear would dissolve.

After the radiation therapy, I developed stabbing pain in the left ear and my throat burned like fire. It was at this time that my first inner wisdom figures appeared during my sessions. They were Native American Indians who told me to listen to the image of the pain and to see what information I could grasp. Part of the message I received was that I would be OK and that my guides were always there for me. I found it was easy to just let the images come on their own without judgment and that I could access them easily. As I continued my inner-work, I found great solace and comfort in the presence of my guides. They were always there to answer my questions and ease my concerns, very often giving me concrete things to do or steps to take. In the very beginning of my encounters with my inner wisdom figures, the information was very simple. Over time the information became more complex as the number of guides grew. Each one had a name and a distinct personality. I discovered who to go to for different issues.

The side effects from my treatments continued. I needed a feeding tube for six weeks because the pain in my throat was so excruciating that I could not swallow. I asked one of my inner wisdom figures how I could heal my throat. By this time, I had developed in imagery a "healing garden" where I would go every time I began my session. The guides in the garden suggested I gather healing herbs-comfrey, echinacea, ruta, arnica, aloe, golden seal and hemlock-and prepare them as a poultice to apply to my throat. I could do it literally or in my imagination. They also suggested I have a dialogue with the pain itself. When I did this I learned that the pain was scared because if it let its defenses down, the pain would be more intense. This gave me some insight into how my body was reacting in response to how I was feeling. I was then told to see an image of my throat as being normal. This proved to be very helpful and I felt myself getting better every day.

Now my healing garden was a place of pure peace, relaxation and comfort to me. It was filled with colors and lush vegetation, beautiful flowers, intricate pathways, ponds and benevolent creatures. I now had five inner wisdom figures to draw upon. It was at this time that I began to deal with my deepest, darkest fears. It became clear that I was afraid of being sick again, of dying and more. Each advisor had a different "energy:" one playful; one wise; one a doctor; one mystical; and one practical. I asked for help with my fears. I was told, "We are all here for you. You'll be fine. We have protected you all your life." They advised me to trust in God and hold this message in my heart to feel calm and peace. Many things were said to me over the years by these beings, always proving to be useful and profound. I found myself beginning to deal with some deep, old issues that, with their help, transformed me in very special ways and allowed me to release old patterns.

My guides and I dealt with childhood issues about how I would get sick a lot to get attention from my parents. When I was five and my ears totally plugged up because of the radiation and I couldn't hear, I became extremely anxious and a feeling of isolation emerged. As I explored this symptom with my inner wisdom figures they helped me see the association between the feeling of isolation as a child and the physical symptom. They explained to me that illness had been a way for me to connect with my parents and was no longer serving me. I saw an image of a dark swamp which was a metaphor of my loneliness as a child. My guides told me to "go through the swamp to the other side." I was assured that I could do it and I would feel better. I didn't have to live in fear of the swamp anymore. Instead of always seeing myself as sickly as I did when I was a child, I was told I needed to change this image of myself and see myself as healthy! Though this sounds simple, it was exactly what I needed to hear at the time.

At the beginning of each session I continued to ask which guide would be the most helpful to work on each question. The one I needed always came forward. I was amazed at the information received as it was always clear, loving and extremely helpful.

I did some "parts work" which was profound. In this work, the strong part of myself was an eagle, who was proud, arrogant, and called the shots. The weak part was a vision of dead flowers in part of my garden. This part of my garden needed more attention and I was told to tend to it as much as I could to bring it back to life. As I did these things, I could feel the transformation happening within me little by little until I felt I had truly transformed my relationship with fear. I felt as if I was put into the burning cauldron and through the burning came the transformation. I don't think I could have ever done this without the help of my guides. I will be forever grateful for their wisdom and guidance and feel blessed to have them with me whenever I need them.

Over the many years since my surgery, I have learned a lot about myself. I see my illness as one of the grandest, most positive things that ever happened to me because I have had the opportunity to change myself in ways I may not have done without the illness. Without imagery I may never have had the opportunity to open the door into my soul that has changed my life for the better.

Imagery for the Relief of Pain

There are many ways to be free. One of them is to transcend reality by imagination, as I try to do.

~ *Anaïs Nin*

Little Green
Inch Worm as Healer

By an imagery guide

*I*t's not very often I keep a client waiting one whole hour! Without going into a long explanation of what happened to cause that to occur, I'll start my story of Mary, who was a very good sport about the long wait. As Mary put it, "My shoulder does not move very well." She recently had left shoulder surgery and had been having difficulty with movement in her shoulder since then. Her injury had occurred when she was carrying heavy boxes while she was helping her daughter move to a new home.

While in the hospital Mary had a session of healing touch that worked very well for her, and she felt very relaxed during that session, so she was excited about the Integrative Imagery process and about experiencing a new healing modality. I explained the use of the inner healer technique as a process that could help explore the limited movement in her left shoulder.

After a guided head-to-toe relaxation with deep breathing and visualizing each major body part relaxed and let go of any tight energy. She relaxed easily and nodded her head as a signal that she was ready to begin. When I invited Mary to go to a special healing place, she found herself in a grass clearing sitting on a red and white checkered blanket with a wicker picnic basket next to her. She could smell the crisp fresh air and feel the cool green grass on her hands. As she described this place, I could almost feel it myself. After giving Mary some time to explore her healing place, I asked her to invite an inner healer to join her there in the special place. She struggled with this a bit and all she could see was a little green inch worm, the kind that pinches up in the middle and then stretches out to move forward. Mary tried to find a different figure, but she could not visualize anything different. She decided to work with the inch worm image and once she made that decision, she accepted the little green inch worm and began quickly to dialogue. Mary described how the inch worm saw her left shoulder as himself. Right now the shoulder was pinched up and could not stretch out. The inch worm said Mary needed to allow her shoulder to stretch out like he did when he moved forward. The worm explained how important Mary's stretching exercises were – even if they hurt a little. Mary spent some time with her inner healer image and invited the image back for a future session. Mary thanked the little inch-worm for all his wisdom and advice and we then finished up the session.

Mary said she felt very rejuvenated after this session. She found it very interesting that the only image that came to her mind was a little green inch worm. Mary could easily see the connection between her shoulder and an inch worm pinched up then stretched out. She confessed she was not doing her range of motion exercises because they hurt a little. The inner healer figure helped her understand how important her exercises were even if they hurt somewhat. She said she would try harder to perform her exercises and was eager to try another session soon.

A True Experience of Transforming Pain

By a student guide

*T*ammy is a fifty-three-year-old woman who I had been seeing for several months. She has been suffering with chronic
pain issues stemming from fibromyalgia. The focus of this session
was to address her pain issue and transform the image of her pain
into a "more workable/tolerable vision."

We had already established a good rapport and trust level and
had discussed the use of guided imagery in dealing with the pain of
her condition. She had previous experience with guided imagery
with the use of a particular audiotape. I began this session by fully
explaining the process, and how drawings are used in this particular imagery modality. At the beginning of this session she described her pain level as an 8 on a scale of 10, with 10 being
extremely painful and 0 being no pain.

We began the session with Tammy coloring the three body
diagrams depicting her pain. The first, "pain at its worst," had very
dark colors encasing her head, torso (front and back) and the outer
aspects of her hips and thighs. The colors were a dark green and
black, the strokes very thick and jagged. The term she used was
"all-encompassing." The second picture, "pain that is tolerable"
was similar in color and placement of the strokes, but the strokes
were not as thick or jagged in nature and she labeled this one "tolerable." The third picture, "pain transformed," she labeled "fantasy" and the colors were a light green and yellow and rather than

thick and jagged the colors radiated out from her body in wispy strokes from each of the areas previously colored in dark tones. There was more space between strokes as well. She felt satisfied with this depiction of her three pain states.

We then began Tammy's descent into a relaxed state by utilizing the agreed upon guided relaxation technique. She was able to establish a level of relaxation and we moved on to inviting her to invoke the image of her special place. She described this as a private, secure little garden with tall fenced walls covered in greenery and ivy. There was the presence of art statuaries and hidden benches and a water fountain. She could hear the water flowing from the fountain, and birds singing, chipmunks scurrying and making noises as they scurried about the garden, and a duck swimming in the fountain. She went to sit on a bench in a little "nook in the corner of the garden." The temperature was mid 70's and the air felt a bit damp to her. She reported feeling safe.

I invited her to recall the first drawing and the image she had created of her "all-encompassing" pain. I suggested that she simply picture it, be aware of it, and not experience it in her body. She could picture her drawing and saw her pain as radiating through her entire body in waves. She was aware of certain spots being very heavy, especially in her shoulders, hips, and back. We did not stay long on this image.

I then guided Tammy to recall the second drawing, the one labeled "tolerable." She was able to shift her image quite easily to the "tolerable" drawing. She stated that there were still "heavy places" but could see the pain change colors and radiate differently. She stated that, "Instead of waves, it washes over me like rays of light, rays of sunshine, warm and comforting-healing." I asked her if she wished to sit with that image for a while and within two minutes she was able to let me know that this was a "nice place to stay," but was ready to move on to the next image.

I again guided her to transform the pain and recall the third drawing labeled "fantasy." She reported that the heavy places didn't exist anymore. It became a "lighter wash, lighter than rays of sunshine, like a light spring shower, or dew drops on the flowers." She stated that the dampness was cleansing for her and that she felt no urgency. She stated that it felt "very odd" to have plenty of time for everything and for doing nothing with no demands on her in one direction or the other. Also that she felt different, "I have no desire to get up and pull weeds, even though there are weeds to pull. It's OK; they'll still be there later. It's peaceful and nice to not have to do anything." I encouraged her to allow the feeling to intensify. She then had an image of putting her hand in the water in the fountain, and getting more comfortable. She began talking to the duck. I asked if it had a message for her. She asked the duck, but wasn't sure if it did. "He's looking at me, not telling me. The more I ask him, he tells me you don't have to talk all the time and it would probably help to listen more. Most of the talking is about fixing and I don't have to fix anything." The duck then jumped in the water and was swimming against Tammy's hand. "He really trusts me; he's letting me feel his feathers. We feel happy." Again I asked her if she wished to simply be with the duck and she did for a minute or two. Then I led her toward closure of the session, suggesting that she could take with her all the learning that this imagery had to offer her.

Upon opening her eyes Tammy stated, "...that was astounding." She briefly talked about how the duck seemed so real and may have more to tell her at a later time. She discussed her feelings about what arose for her during the session. She was able to express her pleasure with actually being able to transform her image and find comfort within her experience. She felt it was not just "an exercise," but rather a true experience of her pain transforming. Although she had begun the session with an 8/10 pain level, she described her pain level after the session as 2 out of 10. She was very pleased with this result. She wanted to write about her experience as a way of helping keep the experience in her mind.

This was my first experience of using this technique. Part of what I learned is the reinforcement of knowing that each person has their own unique wisdom and by facilitating in a non-intrusive, smooth manner, this wisdom comes so naturally. I learned how to gently inquire and step out of the way. It is not about my own ego, but rather a process of releasing my ego in order to be present to the client's process.

A Bough Heavy with Snow

By a student guide

*D*enise is a forty-seven-year-old female, the mother of four young daughters, who works part time as a preschool assistant. She came to see me describing pain in her right elbow radiating down her arm on specific movements. She could not identify the cause of the pain, stating that it just seemed to "appear one day." She said that she tried to ignore the pain and let it take its course, but it had persisted over the last 6 weeks and was starting to interfere with her functioning in daily life. She said that she had not seen a doctor yet but has tried to ice it and take anti-inflammatory drugs to treat it herself in the last week. Denise was not familiar with Integrative Imagery, so I explained the basic process and answered her questions. I suggested a specific technique called "working with an image" that I thought might be helpful for her problem and she agreed to try it.

I asked her to think a minute and try to be as specific as she could about the imaging and what she would like her image to represent. She quickly said that she would like to invite an image to form that would represent her "right elbow pain" or more simply her "elbow pain." The client did not know much about relaxation techniques, so I explained how I would guide her along during the first phase of the imagery session, using deep breathing and progressive muscle relaxation to help her relax. I also suggested we add another basic imaging technique to the relaxation stage called "going to a special place." I explained that imagining a very peaceful, sacred place in nature could work to help her relax further. I also mentioned that "a special place" could also be very useful in creating the environment for inviting an image to form of her "elbow pain." She gestured that she understood and joked that she couldn't wait to "get there."

I started the session by suggesting that she take a couple of deep cleansing breaths and then guided her through progressive muscle relaxation. I asked her to let me know with a nod of her head when she felt relaxed and ready to move on. After a few moments, she nodded and I suggested that when she was ready to allow an image to form of a special place where she felt safe and relaxed. She quickly began to describe a wooded path. She said that it was near her home and she was walking down it with her dog, who was running happily ahead of her. It was winter and the woods were covered with snow, which felt fresh and still. She said that beyond the woods she could see peaceful hills and streams. She described it as a beautiful setting and remarked that she felt "filled-up" and "peaceful." After a few moments to allow her to savor that peaceful feeling, I suggested that she allow an image to form that might represent her "elbow pain".

She began to describe the bough of a large pine tree next to her in the forest. The bough was heavy with snow and looked like it was ready to crack off. I asked her if there was anything else and she said that the bough was very green and fragrant and looked like it was strained. I asked if she thought this image represented the "elbow pain" and she said "yes." I asked her how she felt and she said that she was awed by the beauty of the healthy green bough underneath, but was distressed by the weight of the snow on the bough and worried that it would crack from the pressure. I asked her if there was anything she wanted to say or do to the bough. She said she wanted to shake the snow off of it so that the bough would be relieved of its burden. I suggested that she could do that if she wanted and she did. She felt relief to see the bough bounce back up to its natural position. I asked her if she had any response or insights from this awareness.

She said that she realized that if she wasn't there to brush the snow off the bough, it would have to endure the heaviness until someone came along to help or until the sun was so warm that it melted the snow. This brought to mind her issue with her elbow pain. The image gave her the insight that if she let her pain "heal naturally," as she had done in the past, without intervention, that it would take too long and may break her "spirit." She said that she is an active and healthy runner, who enjoys her body and does not like the idea of loosing her spirit. She said she thinks that she is fighting treatment because she feels that if she "succumbs" to it, it would mean that she is aging and loosing control of her body. Having seen the strain on the bough, she realized that she needed to reconsider her idea of "ignoring her pain." Instead, she needs to explore other treatment options or she risks the possibility that her elbow may break down further. The client understood what this meant. I then reminded her that our time was almost up and suggested that she might look around again to see if there was anything else she wanted to say or do before she left. I gently suggested that if it felt right, she might want to thank the image for coming and she could revisit this place and image again in the future if she needed to. She smiled and indicated with a nod that she was ready to come back to the energy of the room. I directed her to gently move her fingers and toes and slowly open her eyes when she was ready.

Although Denise was new to the whole process of relaxation and imagery, I think she did well in clarifying the issues around her elbow pain. She was surprised by her concerns about the aging process. She acknowledged that the session helped her realize that she was resistant about attending to her elbow pain because she wanted her body to perform in the "self-healing" mode as it had always done in the past. She recognized that after 6 weeks of pain without relief, she needed to consider a different approach. We talked about the idea of "natural healing" and I explained that she could still incorporate and count on this concept. We talked about how the body does have a self-healing system that is effective in most situations, but it's important to recognize that it sometimes needs support. I suggested that she have a health professional evaluate her pain, listen to the recommendations for treatment and request natural healing methods. She liked the idea and said that she thought she would do this. She brought up the idea of finding a symbol, such as a picture of a small, snow covered tree to add to her home altar to remind her of the insights she gained in this process.

Better than Drugs!

By an imagery guide

*B*etty is a middle-aged woman with a long, long history of substance abuse who is also HIV-positive. She has been clean and sober for several years but had been having trouble with the side effects of medications for both her HIV and her chronic liver disease. She came to me for help with stress management and to learn techniques that would assist her in reducing or omitting the need for pain medications. In our very first session she found her special place which was a grotto with cool running water. She immersed herself in this cool water to relax her body. She used this often to help deal with the physical discomfort of her conditions. In subsequent sessions she used the "transforming pain" technique to ease physical symptoms that were painful, especially the day after her weekly Interferon injections.

As time went on she met and consulted with Hannah, her Inner Wisdom figure. Hannah was a little, short and wrinkly old woman who wore a big cloak. Hannah offered both support and reassurance to Betty that her physical discomfort was a direct result of the medications. Hannah's cool hands offered relief for this pain and discomfort. In time Betty integrated her imagery sessions into her real life by physically getting into a cool tub of water, lighting candles and listening to soft music. Betty would listen to tapes made during our sessions or practice her own imagery experience.

In time, Betty was ready to begin dealing with the emotional discomfort of her conditions and found herself in a cozy library with books she could consult. One of the books she used was entitled <u>Tolerance</u>; the other <u>Patience</u>. Betty's description of these books went like this: "<u>Patience</u> is not well used or read and it looks as if it has not been opened very often. This is not a very big book but it feels heavy and substantial. It has thick pages and soft leather on the outside. <u>Tolerance</u> is bigger and more dog-eared and maybe used a lot more. The back of the book is more well-read than the front half as indicated by the dog-eared pages. This book feels familiar to me and I do not have to read it to know what is inside. Just by holding it I remember what is inside. It feels warm."

By exploring these imaginary books Betty was able to let go of the intensity of her emotional challenges and "lighten up" the pictures, which resulted in her lightening up emotionally. Perhaps the biggest help to Betty has been her ability to refrain from using pain medication which she views as a high risk for her due to her years as a heroin addict. She feels that the techniques she has learned have saved her life and allows her to function as normally as possible for someone in her situation. She feels that the ability to relax and use her mind to control her physical and emotional feelings is "a miracle." She pretty much summed it up for herself in one of our early sessions. As she was being guided back to the present, she gently opened her eyes, a beautiful peaceful smile broke out on her face and she quietly stated, "That's almost as good as heroin."

Numbing the Pain Away

By a student guide

Kathryn is a seventy-six-year-old woman who had recently taken a fall and had fractured her left arm just below the elbow. She was in a significant amount of pain because her arm could not be put in a cast. Her doctor had placed it in a sling instead, which allowed some movement and therefore an increase in the pain. She had no experience with imagery at all, but was quite open to anything that could help reduce her pain level. I inquired about her pain level at the beginning of the session. She rated it as a 4 on a scale of 1 to 10, with 10 being extremely painful and 1 being no pain at all.

I suggested Kathryn take a few deep breaths and proceeded to lead her in the relaxation exercise. She responded well and let me know when she was ready to move onto the next step. I directed her to imagine there was a bucket full of ice cold water next to her on her right side. I had her imagine all the details of the bucket. She saw an old fashioned wooden bucket with a handle. It was filled with "crystal clear water." I invited her to add a magic ingredient to the water to increase its ability to numb her hand as she submerged it slowly in the imaginary ice cold water in the bucket. She actually could sense her hand getting cold as she did the imagery. I reminded her that the rest of her body was warm and relaxed. When her hand got to the point of being as cold as it could get I invited her to remove her right hand and place it on her left arm where she was feeling the pain. She placed her "numbed" hand on her broken arm and held it for about five minutes. During those few minutes, I encouraged her to allow the feeling of numbness to transfer into her left arm so that she could soak in all the numbing relief. She could actually feel the pain dissolving underneath her hand. When she was finished soaking in all the numbing relief, I then invited her to bring her focus back to the present. After taking a few deep breaths she opened her eyes. She was quite amazed that this helped. After the imagery session she rated her pain as 1 out of 10.

This imagery session went very smoothly for Kathryn. She responded well and was quite amazed at her ability to do this and have it make such a difference in her level of pain and discomfort. What was particularly fun about this is that she now has a skill that she can use for herself that makes a big difference in her healing process. She told me a few weeks later that she had tried it several times on her own and it had worked well those times as well. Her physician was quite impressed with how well and quickly she healed from this fracture.

Playing with Flipper

By a student guide

At 55, Rosie has been suffering with fibromyalgia, a painful muscular weakness that is very debilitating. She is in considerable pain and would like to connect with that wise healing part of herself. She would like an inner healer to help her with the pain in her muscles and joints. We discussed the importance of finding a healing place and calling forth an inner healer. Other than the fibromyalgia, Rosie has no other medical conditions.

To begin the session, I facilitated a head-to-toe relaxation and when Rosie relaxed she signaled to me with a gentle nod of her head.

I began, "As your body remains comfortable and relaxed, imagine yourself in a special healing place, a place that is most suited for you. Let me know when you are there and begin to describe what it is like."

"I am in the water in Hawaii. I feel so relaxed. I can hear the gentle breeze rustling in the palm fronds. The sun feels so warm. My eyes are closed and I feel like I am drifting up and down---rocking---like in a cradle."

"Allow yourself to bask in this relaxation in the buoyant water with the warm sun. When you are ready, allow an image to appear of an inner healer, one that is wise, loving and possesses the healing power that is needed to decrease the pain in your joints and muscles."

"I hear him. He is a dolphin. He just playfully splashed me."

"Tell me more about this playful dolphin. Does he have a name?"

"Yes, it's Flipper. He has ancient wisdom. He is so playful. He feels smooth. I'm touching his side. He is so, so calm. Whoops! There he goes. He just did a spin. He is a spinnaker dolphin." "Ask him if he is willing to help you in your healing."

"Yes, he says the pain will go away when I become more playful."

Some time passed…

I asked, "What is happening?"

"I'm spinning around and around with Flipper. The spinning is sending tingling through my whole body."

"Stay with it."

"I am so relaxed….calm….peaceful."

A few minutes passed,

I gently asked, "Is there anything else that needs to happen?"

"No, Flipper says that's enough for one day. 'Just be playful!' He is gone."

"Take a moment to thank yourself and wave goodbye and thank Flipper, knowing that you can come back here any time. When you are done gently bring yourself back to the room. Let yourself become aware of the sounds around you, the couch beneath you and open your eyes feeling awake and alert." After the session, Rosie and I talked a bit.

I inquired, "How are you feeling?"

"I have never felt so relaxed and calm in my life."

"Did you gain any insights during your imagery experience?"

"Yes, to be more playful. I know now that I need to take the time to really relax. I feel like I have less pain right now. I would like to do this again.

Rosie is a dear friend and she truly experienced pain relief during this one session.

Imagery with Kids

One of the virtues of being very young is that you don't let the facts get in the way of your imagination.

~ Sam Levenson

Mystic Knows the Song

By a student guide

*C*hristine is a 5th grade student who participates in many extra-curricular activities. The activities include soccer, piano, horseback riding, cello, and Girl Scouts. She is feeling a bit over-whelmed and anxious because she has signed up to perform in a variety show for the 5th grade. Out of 200 students she is the only one that has agreed to perform a solo song. This is the day of the performance and she is feeling "scared that she will not remember the lyrics." She has had many sessions of imagery and is quite comfortable with the process. She thinks that she is a "seeing, hearing, and touching" processor (visual, auditory and kinesthetic) and wants help with "only breathing for relaxation." We discuss about going to a special, safe, favorite place. She is very specific in request for an image of Inner Wisdom. She wants an image to come and help her with her performance.

Christine quickly relaxed using the "balloon breath" I learned from Dr. Charlotte Reznick who specializes in working with chil-dren. Our session went as follows:

"We are going to begin by placing your hands on your tummy and taking a nice deep breath and letting yourself relax. Begin to imagine your tummy is like a balloon and when you breathe in your tummy gets a little bit larger and fills with the air you breathe in. When you breathe out all that air releases and goes away. Take a nice deep breath in (count 1-2-3). Hold it and let go (count 1-2-3)."

We did a few short minutes of the breathing and she signaled with a nod that she was relaxed. Our session continued:

"While your body remains very relaxed and comfortable begin to imagine yourself in your favorite, special, safe place. It can be a place you have been before or a new place in your imagination, a place where you can meet a wise, knowing part of yourself. Begin to describe what you see, smell, feel and hear in this place."

"I am at the beach in Hawaii. The turtles are all around me. The water is so warm and clear. I can see for miles. I am swimming after the fish and the turtles are right on my side. I love it here. I am alone but not really--all of my sea friends are here. Squirrel is here. (Squirrel is a guide from a previous imagery session that helped Christine with a math test). Lou Shing is here." (Lou Shing is "the blue dragon that protects from humiliation," another guide from a previous imagery session.) Dolphin is here (an imaginary friend from a past imagery session who is always with her).

"How are you feeling?"

"I feel great. I love it here."

"Take a moment to really enjoy this beautiful place at the beach. When you are ready invite an image that represents your Inner Wisdom--one that is wise, loving, knowledgeable, a part of you that knows all the lyrics and music to your song."

"I hear her. She is on the shore. She is so beautiful."

"Go on."

"She is a sparkling white unicorn. She is watching me. She seems to be smiling. Her name is Mystic."

"Tell me more about Mystic. What else do you notice?"

"She is kind. She said I can climb up on her back."

Some time passes and I ask, "What is happening?"

"We are flying all over the beach. I am on her back."

"Is Mystic an image of an animal that knows all the lyrics and music to your song?"

"Yes, she was singing my song when I first saw her."

"Do you think that you could ask Mystic if she could be with you during your performance to help you remember your song?"

"Yes, she said that she could be with me."

"Take a moment to thank Mystic and tell her you will see her at the concert or whenever you want. When you are ready, come back and begin to feel the bed beneath you, slowly open your eyes."

When the session was over, I asked Christine how she was feeling. She stated that she felt less nervous about the performance and she willingly drew a picture of Mystic for herself.

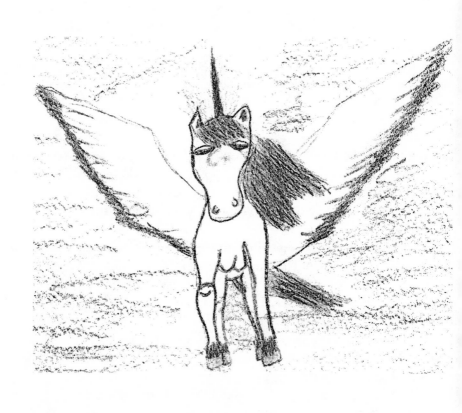

Sleeping in My Own Bed

By a student guide

*W*endy is a five-year-old who is afraid to sleep by herself, so I used the "transforming pain" technique and substituted "fear" for "pain." This is a description of a first session in a probably on-going process to help Wendy acquire the skills she needs to sleep alone in her own bed.

In the "transforming fear" technique we used three pictures we entitled "frightened," "tiny frightened," and "not frightened" to help Wendy transform her experience of fear. In the first picture, Wendy said she drew brown legs because "when Mommy wants me to sleep in my own bed my legs start to shake and feel weak." "My tummy is red because it gets all tied up in knots. The blond hair and red brain are for fun." In the second picture Wendy described, "my feet are purple because only my feet shake and curl under when Mommy wants me to sleep in my own bed. My head is yellow because my head shakes a little, too. The red hair is just for fun." Of the third picture Wendy said, "my green arms feel lazy and relaxed. The purple neck is soft and relaxed. The brown hair is for fun."

Wendy is very visual and described interesting observations. In the first picture (at her most frightened) she saw herself rolling into a little ball, rolling down the stairs into a small hiding place when her Mommy asked her to try sleeping alone. When she felt "tiny frightened," she pictured herself climbing a tree and learning how to fly. I encouraged her to continue feeling free and relaxed and asked her to picture the third drawing ("not frightened"). Wendy described a feeling of strength with a thick gray tree trunk that was so strong not even thunder storms could blow it down. When I asked Wendy how she could bring this thought and feeling into her mind again, she said that she could go into her "thinking corner," close her eyes and picture a big tall gray tree trunk.

Wendy thought the experience was very fun and seemed more interested in doing imagery again rather than learning to sleep alone. We talked about how Mommy was trying to help her feel strong like the big gray tree trunk and how she could use that feeling for many situations in life. Wendy was very receptive to this and we agreed to try the relaxation process and by calling back some images when she was lying in her own bed at night. Most nights, Wendy now sleeps safely in her own bed using the image of the big tree.

From Frightened
to Fearless

By a student guide

*E*van is a very introverted six-year-old child who is anxious and self-conscious in new and crowded places. This anxiety is manifested in picking the skin around both thumbnails and biting a few of his fingernails. He sometimes picks at scabs that often appear around the time of school pictures or Christmas card pictures. This is a description of a first session of Integrative Imagery that will hopefully become an ongoing process of learning better ways to express his fears and anxieties.

I asked Evan first to draw a picture of his fear/anxiety at its worst. In the first picture, which we entitled "frightened," Evan drew red which he said represented his blood circulating. A green heart indicated that he was frightened. A purple brain represented his thinking about picking his skin and biting his nails. Green on the arms represented his feeling frightened and wanting to pick.

A second drawing we entitled "hardly frightened." In his picture, Evan drew a red heart connected to a red brain which represented his finding a new friend. Because he felt happy he did not feel the need to bite his nails ever again. On the right side of the picture he drew green veins and a green heart which meant he was sad because he lost his friend.

The third picture, entitled "not frightened," represented the ideal (no fear or anxiety). Evan drew a red heart and veins leading to green and a purple brain which represented extreme happiness because he found lots of friends and felt he would never need to bite his fingernails again.

It was challenging to guide Evan through this process. His self-conscious nature made it difficult to go through the three pictures and explore and observe his feelings. With the first picture he described a "weird" feeling inside that made him want to hide in his room. He felt people were looking at him and didn't like him. In working with the second picture, we tried to work on observing rather than feeling or experiencing, but Evan kept going back to his experience of feeling better when he has a friend. The third picture (when he imagined not being frightened at all) he described feeling good when he reads a book or does an activity.

So, we pulled together the idea of reading with an adult when Evan was starting to feel frightened about something to help get his mind off of his fear. This was linked with a physical cue (pressing his fingers together gently) to help empower him to make the frightened feeling go away.

This was an illuminating experience for me, as Evan seemed distracted and very fidgety during the whole process. Yet, in the evaluation he remembered everything and was very talkative. He was excited about reading to help him get over his fears and showed how he would work on pressing his fingers together rather than picking or biting his nails. It seemed he got more out of the session than I was aware of at the time.

Over the many months since Evan learned this technique, he has successfully replaced the nail picking with his physical cue of pressing his fingers together. This experience helped me realize how people, even children, can take what they need from an imagery experience in their own way !

Blue Dragon Brings Relaxation and Freedom

By a student guide

*H*ana is a sweet, little ten-year-old girl who has been on many different medications for asthma. For the past three months she has had a chronic cough, which is disturbing for her, especially at school. She would like to go to school and not cough. Right now the only things that bring her some relief are drinking water and taking her medicine. As I talked to Hana, she told me that on a scale of 0 to 10, with 0 being no cough and 10 being a continuous cough, her present discomfort level is a 5. After we discussed some possible imagery techniques, she chose "transforming pain or discomfort" saying, "I would like to know what it feels like not to cough." Her choice seemed wise, as this technique has the potential to create a template for Hana's mind and body to actually decrease or dissipate her cough completely.

I explained that we would be drawing three pictures of her perception of the discomfort of the cough. The first picture would be the cough at its "worst," the second picture would be the cough at its "least," and the third picture would be the cough completely "gone." Hana, however, had other ideas. She had a little trouble with the concept of the cough at its "least," saying, "I either have the cough or not. I only want to draw two pictures – 'cough' and 'no cough'." She said she believed it could be gone permanently. We agreed that after she drew the first picture of "cough" I would help her to do a relaxation technique then recall the picture in her imagination. Then I would invite her to transform the picture of "cough" into a picture of "no cough."

Our session proceeded as we had planned. Hana relaxed quickly and was able to recall her picture of "cough" in her mind's eye. I encouraged her to observe the image and describe her feelings.

"I feel irritated. The cough irritates me." She began to cough.

I asked, "Are you feeling it or observing it? Just watch the picture as if it were on a TV and begin to describe to me what you see."

"I'm watching the picture now (the cough had subsided). There is a black widow spider hanging from her baby finger. She is deathly afraid of spiders and she hates centipedes. She is irritated. Marissa irritates her. James irritates her. Madeline irritates her. And homework somewhat irritates her. She is dressed in black because she is sad. There are crosses and RIP sign because it feels like Death."

"Are you still observing or feeling?"

"I'm watching. Her hair is frizzy. I hate that she has ripples of fat on her stomach. The scars are the cuts on her body the cough has made."

I told her to take a deep breath and to let go of her cough and to transform that image to the second drawing of the image without the cough. Then I asked her to describe it to me and to tell me how she felt.

Her eyes opened briefly. She said, "I feel free-- so free. I'm not scared. I can breathe easily." She then began to describe the transformed picture she saw in her mind's eye. "She is glowing like an angel. She has halos above her head and all her favorite animals are next to her. They all can fly. There is my flying pig, my flying cow and my magical flying unicorn. The black widow spider has turned into a butterfly. There is a beautiful blue dragon flying above her to protect her. She is wearing light blue because it is the color of the ocean and it feels cool and comfortable."

"Hana, how are you feeling now?"

"I am feeling so relaxed and I am not coughing. I feel so free."

"Take a moment and pay close attention to how your body feels right now."

"I feel so relaxed and free. I don't feel like coughing anymore."

"Allow yourself to take a few minutes and really feel this relaxation without the cough."

After a few minutes I asked her, "Is there something you can bring back with you from this image that will help remind you of this relaxed feeling?"

"Yes, I will bring back the blue dragon."

"Ask the blue dragon if it would be willing to come back with you to remind you of this feeling of relaxation and freedom."

"Yes, he will."

"Take a moment more to really feel this relaxation and freedom. If you would like, say thank you to the dragon, angel, unicorn or anyone else.

"I said thank you to all of them. I'm done."

In the discussion following the imagery, I encouraged Hana to look at her drawings. She declined to add or change any image. She said that she felt so much happier and more relaxed now that she was not coughing. I asked her if she thought she could use the "no cough" image that she had drawn. She replied that all she had to do was "imagine." She surprised me by asking for some paper and pen. She proceeded to write the following story:

A Different Kind of Hero
written by Hana

Once there was a princess who had everything she could possibly dream of, except freedom. She loved her parents very much but she wanted more. She wanted to travel the Universe and have adventures.

She was near her lake filled with emerald green lily pads and golden fish watching the snowy feather swan swim gracefully across the water. She imagined herself swimming in a dark, cool, crystal-clear ocean looking for buried treasure when she saw a poor woman selling bread. The princess was so kind she bought some. The poor woman thanked her and gave her some bread.

As the princess was walking away the woman asked her, "why are you so miserable?'

The princess said, "I have no freedom."

The poor woman looked confused. "Why do you say that," said the woman. "Of course you have freedom."

"No, I don't," said the princess. "I'm stuck here between these four gray cold stone walls."

"That is the way you see it," said the woman. "What were you thinking of just then?"

The princess told her and then a huge smile spread across the woman's face and she spoke these ten words, "You can go anywhere you want when you imagine it."

Just then a thought struck the princess –"the old woman is right." So, she closed her eyes and imagined a beautiful, peaceful meadow covered in ruby red roses and in the center was a white dove. When the princess was done, she opened her eyes so she could thank the woman, but she was gone.

The Moral

Imagination can take you anywhere and you can do anything. Therefore, you can be your own hero every day.

This session proved to be dramatically successful. Hana went off all medications except one, and now, after five months, is medication-free with no cough.

The previous stories are just some of the many amazing tales that reflect the power of the human spirit. As described in the introduction, the different Integrative Imagery techniques give the structure to this process of creativity and healing. Something profound happens when we go to that deep knowing place beyond ordinary consciousness. The imagery process then becomes the evolving story that is revealed to the imager, transforming metaphor into reality. Emmett Miller, MD describes it this way: "The storyteller, the image maker, is the true healer. At both a personal and a global level, our future will be determined by our ability to be responsible and wise with the stories we tell ourselves. For as we imagine, so we will become."

Section Three:
The Ripple Effect

Go confidently in the direction of your dreams. Live the life you have imagined.

~ Henry David Thoreau

*I*n this section we present seven diverse samplings of the many creative ways people are applying Integrative Imagery in their careers. The possibilities are infinite.

Time and time again, professionals involved in the Beyond Ordinary Nursing Certificate Program in Imagery and those participating in the Integrative Imagery process speak about the personal transformation and the life-changing experiences that occur for them. Dreams are ignited. New careers involving imagery are imagined. Incorporating Integrative Imagery into a current healthcare practice enriches that practice. As the graduates of the program reflect upon the deep inner work they have discovered, they return to their communities to share and expand the healing effects of this work.

In Qigong (an ancient Chinese body movement and energy practice) one form, called "Pebble in the Lake" eloquently represents this. A person stands in a relaxed posture and visualizes dropping a simple pebble into the calm surface of a lake. Then he drops the focus of his attention deep into the core of the body. As the image of the pebble settles into the water, it creates concentric rings on the surface of the water that spreads out in ever-widening circles, originating from the center. There is a simultaneous deepening and expansion that keeps continuing. This is the ripple effect.

This natural principle has been a guiding force for the co-founders of BON on our own personal journeys and a recurrent theme as this work is shared with others in the world. The ripples of Integrative Imagery are real and tangible. The following examples are the living proof of this magical ripple effect in real life.

A Dream-
Only an Image Away

By an imagery client

My name is Francesca. My first imagery session was in December 1996. I was caring for my terminally ill mother in my home, trying to work full-time in an abusive job, carrying a huge financial burden, was in a challenging relationship, and had minimal support from family and friends. I was overwhelmed, having trouble remembering things, depressed, experiencing nightmares and suffering from high blood pressure due to the burden I was carrying.

Many issues were addressed during the six months I actively worked with an Integrative Imagery practitioner. In the nine years that have followed, a dream that had resurfaced during those imagery sessions continued to live in my heart and got me through many difficult challenges as I was putting my life back together. When I felt devastated, angry and in deep grief over my mother's death, the dream came back to me. Every time I got knocked off the ladder I got back on, using imagery tools to stay focused on an inner strength and the belief that I could succeed in bringing the dream to reality. I could see it, taste it and touch it.

My dream was to create my own business that reflected my love for beauty and art, a retail store that would be a "sensorama" with a French flavor that specialized in invitations and events. I created a storyboard in my mind's eye; touching and feeling the textures of the merchandise, seeing the colors and experiencing them used by customers. I would then actually buy materials that I could touch and hold on to in my "real world." I did research and studied vendors that I would like to work with and envisioned myself inside my store surrounded by loveliness and the contentment of my achievement.

Ten years to the month after my first imagery session, my store was created in a room in my home. Little did I know that my imagery would one day encompass my mother's spirit. The room had been my mother's bedroom and most of the authentic antique furniture belonged to her. The butter-yellow walls, the topiary painting on the door, the chandelier lighting, the fabrics, and the paper are all are exactly as I pictured them on my imaginary storyboard.

I am busy at work with my business, experiencing the fulfillment of my dreams and helping others realize their own by sharing my own journey. The dream has materialized and the imagery is going beyond the small room into an enhancement of ideas and visions. My imagery is alive and well and continues to help me grow into the future.

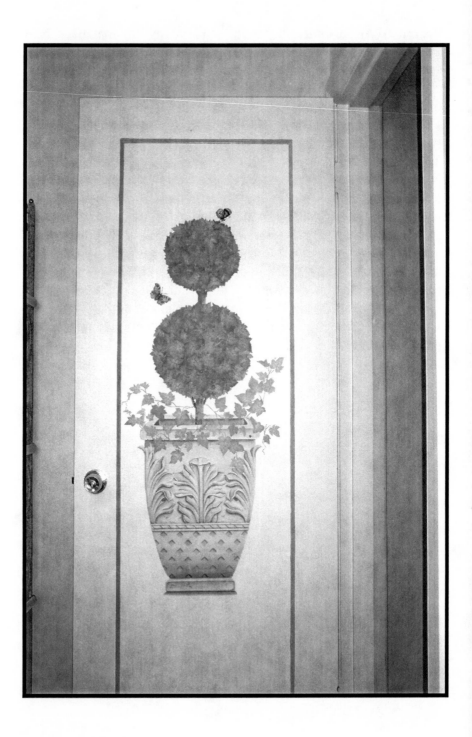

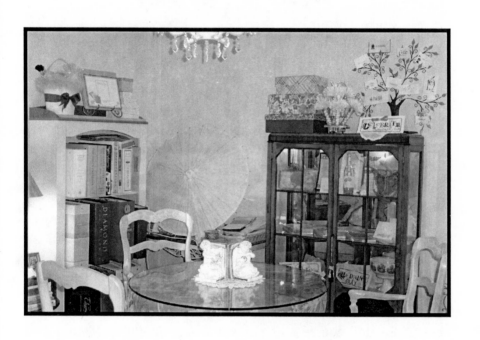

Transforming Images into Reality

By an imagery practitioner

*T*he fury of ideas galloping through my head did not match the sluggish pace of rush hour traffic. But as my foot was alternating impatiently between the pedals, I realized that I was weighing my ideas on a similar scale-gas on one side and brakes on the other. How would they be received?

The intense desire to do something extraordinary in the second half of my life fueled and inspired my dreams. But the biggest barricade I encountered was my own skepticism. It blocked me at almost every turn, challenging me to meet it head on and find a way to overcome it. As I exited the freeway, I began to reflect on my acceptance and invitation to Beyond Ordinary Nursing's Integrative Imagery program. The thrill and gratitude of having been included in this course had not yet faded. Initially, when I first enrolled, the program was offered only to nurses and health professionals. I felt so fortunate to have been the exception to that rule. Having already completed Phase I and II, I was about to begin Phase III. As an artist, part of my adventure had become discovering a way to use my newly acquired imagery skills in the field of graphic design. Exploring that potential seemed powerful and limitless.

I stepped out of the car feeling both excited and anxious at the anticipation of expressing my ideas to the Phase III group. Determined, I resolved to take some deep breaths and shake off any remaining doubt. I walked into the room where the initial exchange of friendly conversation and welcoming smiles helped calm my nerves. The group slowly quieted down for our meeting to begin. And within a few minutes, individuals started sharing experiences that had occurred in their lives during our three-month break. When my turn finally came, I gathered the courage to explain the process I had envisioned. I wanted to help people create their own business identities, logos, and product designs using imagery as the foundation. Following each imagery session, clients would be asked to sketch the images that arose in colored pen, even if they appeared rudimentary or simple on paper. Those simple illustrations and the sensory information gathered during our sessions together would be articulated into computer design software for a finished graphic design. Could it work?

The group responded to my idea with overwhelming enthusiasm and I felt assured that I was headed in the right direction. All the doubt and uncertainty I had been holding suddenly washed away. They gave me the confidence that I needed to move forward and ask my first client if she would be willing to try this method to create her product design. She wholeheartedly agreed.

After completing two imagery sessions with my client, the composition for her logo design became clear. The impressions from her imagery experiences and rough drawings translated beautifully into computer illustrator software. It was a striking design. Not only was it uniquely hers, it embodied what she wanted her business to project into the community and the world.

For myself, I discovered that I had been building my own roadblock, cemented with criticism and self-doubt. I had unwittingly barred myself from moving forward. But when I finally left the inner critic at the door I felt confident and free to blend two fields that I love: imagery and graphic design. The beautiful images that people hold inside never cease to amaze me and each image has a wonderful story to tell. I am honored to hold that space for clients as those images develop. Translating the pictures in their imaginations into visual art is an incredible experience.

Accessing Financial Wisdom Through Imagery

By an imagery practitioner

*I*magery has been a thread running through my life as long as I can remember. Today, it's part of the work I do in the world as a financial counselor and coach. When people think of money they mostly think of numbers, calculators and the left-brain. Indeed this is a vital part of any financial process.

It's surprising for people to learn that the right-brain takes on just as vital a role in one's financial life. It's the right brain that holds the wisdom of a client's belief system. This wisdom can be accessed by calling forth images. These images can take the shape of financial advisors; head vs. heart mediators; or the polarized images of "lack" and its opposite, "abundance."

By accessing images, clients can gain insight into unconscious belief systems they may be acting out in their financial lives or unlock understanding about beliefs and behaviors regarding money. When clients understand why and how they create blocks to abundance, they can then do something about that. They can gain insight into their true needs and begin to bring to themselves the money they want to support these needs. Working together with both numbers and images creates a powerful combination for the client. It is the equivalent of the left and right brain in conversation-listening, negotiating and making decisions for their highest good.

Sometimes, stories are the best examples. Using the imagery technique of "polarity work" (also called "parts work") one of my clients chose to access an image of "lack" and an image of "abundance."

Her image of "lack" was a crusted gnarly toothless sailor that hadn't had a bath in months and who was wearing torn and tattered clothes. His name was "Curly." Curly worked hard his entire life. His knuckles were raw, bleeding and red. His fingernails were dirty. His life energy was dim. He walked folded over as if carrying a heavy burden on his back. His bloodshot eyes looked down at the ground. Oddly, he sported a wide grin on his wrinkled face. When asked what message he had to deliver, he stated, "I'm tired, I want to retire."

When accessing an image of "abundance," a figure named "Pippee" appeared in my client's mind's eye. She had long red pigtails that swayed in the wind. Her spirit was light and bouncy and filled with the energy of joy. She seemed animated in her play, was light-hearted and seemed ready to see the humor in things. When any problem presented itself, Pippee laughed and let solutions come forth rather than forcing or working hard to find the answers. Her motto was "relax and let go."

Through the use of imagery, this client found a way to give permission to Curly to slow down, stop working and actually retire. In the "real" physical world, using the image of Curly gave the client the fortitude to create change by slowing down and working part-time. When she did, her life became more abundant and lively with the energy of Pippee. Although this client brought in less money in a given month, she was able to live within her means, save, and breathe life into her dreams-- all at the same time. She didn't fritter money away anymore; she became more conscious of it and became more financially astute. She found more enjoyment in being with friends than she did in buying more things for her home. Working less created a balance in her life. For the first time ever, she experienced "space" in her day between her activities. She experienced inner joy by playing in her garden and taking her dog for walks. Solutions to problems seemed to flow effortlessly to her. She was able to improvise and create.

I feel blessed to be doing this work, helping people to overcome fears, worries and anxiety about money and assisting them to shift to a place of abundance in their lives. In a former life I was an intensive care nurse, today I am a financial coach! In order for this transformation to have happened in my own life, I employed my imagination to help me create the life I desired. I cut pictures out of magazines that "spoke to dreams" and created a vision board that I could see every day. I looked at the images that held my dreams and desires. After awhile I internalized these images and made them real.

When I felt fear in moving forward in a new direction, I used imagery to help me move through the fear, to unlock the "stuck" parts of myself. I conversed with these parts of myself and encouraged them so they would feel safe moving forward. Imagery helped me discover my true needs, passions and desires. By having access to the information through the imagery process I was empowered to move into greater congruency in my own life. I was able to let go of what no longer worked and feed my spirit to embrace new opportunities. I was able to live with uncertainty and stay in the mystery of life, because I believed new images would appear. I just needed to be present to see them when they did.

I believe images and the information the images offer are messages from our "highest self," our true divine nature. In the words of William Arthur Ward, "If we can imagine it, we can achieve it; if we can dream it, we can become it." Imagery has been a spiritual journey for me, connecting me to my highest self and to my source energy! It is a gift for which I'm truly thankful.

Confessions of a
Reluctant Therapist

By an imagery practitioner

I am the reluctant therapist. I didn't sit around as a kid and dream that someday I would grow up and save people's lives by talking them in or out of things. In fact, my career started as a teacher and I cannot tell you why I ever gave that up. I found myself getting a master's in social work and viola! I am a therapist. Some days, I still can't believe that people actually pay me for this. I really love what I do and I find that gratitude continually swells in my soul when I know that I am going to work. How many people can actually say that? I am one of the truly blessed "lucky ones."

However, it wasn't always this way. I think I had to find the "therapy skin" in which to be comfortable. And that is where imagery comes in. Let me tell you the story of how imagery changed my life and the lives of the many clients I see. But mostly, this story is about how imagery made therapy fun for me and since it was fun and interesting for me, I could transfer that to the people that I see.

It was like any other day, really. I found myself going to a two-day conference, dreading it. I had been in private practice for nearly two years and I was already itching to get out of it. Maybe I would get another government job, I dreamed. Or maybe I would grow up and become a famous journalist traveling the world reporting murder and mayhem. I wanted action and excitement and frankly sitting day after day and listening to people's issues did not do it for me. I dutifully acted as a therapist, as I had been taught to do in school. I was passive and non-interactive. I would nod my head and say the occasionally "huh" and "oh" and "tell me about that" whenever it was appropriate. And I was bored, bored, and more bored.

Here I am at the imagery conference. Two more boring days listening to two speakers drone on and on. At least I would get lots of continuing education hours and I could sit in the back and draw funny faces to keep me amused. If you haven't guessed already, I am easily bored. So, I settled down with my yellow note pad and waited, already deciding to draw a strange looking man sitting just ahead of me. And then, the speaker came to the podium. I was instantly hooked. And I mean instantly.

The conference went on for the two days but it just flew by for me. I was like a thirsty person who needed water desperately and finally some kind being came along and fed me clear, icy, streaming water. This was it. This was what was missing in my "boring" practice. I listened to story after story from the speakers about the power of imagery to change lives and to change minds. It was *true*. I knew it deep, deep in my spirit. I was and always have been an imaginative person. I image everything. I have little plays that go on in my head all the time. I had an imaginary friend as a child named "Freddy."

When I was a waterfront co-director for three summers at a camp for inner-city kids in New York and New Jersey, I made swimming lessons creative and full of imaginary "water beings." The kids loved it and they learned to overcome their fear of water and swim because of the power of the imagination. But I had not transferred that super-creative, imaginative side to my therapy. Instead, I let my degrees and education get in the way. But that was about to change.

I went back to my practice a "new" person. Or maybe I became the person I always was. I started using imagery immediately although I look back now and am positively horrified at how many mistakes I made. My patients didn't seem to notice. They loved it. They began to tell their friends about the "wacky mind stuff" that I was doing and I had people come to see for themselves what all the fuss was about.

The expression "change your mind, change your life" really is appropriate for the way that imagery revolutionized my practice. Through the power of imagery I "changed" my mind and went back to being who I was rather than what graduate school tried to make me. Imagery changes people's minds. Imagery changes people's lives.

And ultimately, isn't that what therapy is all about?

Blending Shamanic Healing with Integrative Imagery

By an imagery practitioner

*I*n some ways, Integrative Imagery could not be more different from Shamanic Healing. Integrative Imagery is very client centered, and one of the major goals is to illicit feelings so that
the client can acknowledge those feelings and gain insight and
awareness. The guide "stays out of the process" and focuses on
facilitating.

In shamanic healing the focus is on the healer, who goes into a
trance state to receive information about the client from the intuitive realm the shamans call the "Middle World." Often, in the
Middle World, power animals come to share information. The
concept is that sometimes people are adversely affected by a
wounding or emotional event that they experienced in their life.
Sometimes they are not aware of this wounding and on an emotional or energetic level it keeps them from true wholeness. The
trained shaman can receive and share information about the
wounding so healing and wholeness can happen.

My interest, as an imagery practitioner of many years and a
new and fascinated practitioner of shamanism, is to marry the two
healing modalities. I find that when used together some amazing
healing occurs. As I continue to blend the two, I have been privi-

leged to be a witness to some very powerful changes through this blending.

One particular client is foremost in my mind. I had been working for a number of years with a gentleman, Jim, whose goal was to retire from an extremely stressful work environment healthy and whole. He had witnessed many of his colleagues succumb to heart attacks, mental breakdowns, or other such devastating symptoms of chronic stress. With that in mind, he had come to see me for acupressure and stress management. Over the years I worked with him we did more than a few Integrative Imagery sessions, so he was comfortable with the process. He was aware that I had been studying ancient healing practices and was open and interested in shamanic healing.

One day Jim came in to the office with a terrible cough and lung congestion. As I was using acupressure points to ease and soothe his congestion, I held my hand over his heart chakra. The room was quiet and peaceful when intuitively I knew to ask silently if Jim had a power animal that would like to make itself known. Immediately, a beautiful white dove appeared in my mind's eye. I continued to hold the heart chakra point and keep the image of the dove in my mind. When I began to move my hand to change to a different acupressure point, I felt an invisible force restrain my hand and heard a voice say, "Not yet!" It was such a surprisingly strong command that I chuckled a bit. Since the room had been so quiet and peaceful, it seemed appropriate to let Jim know why I had chuckled. I shared my vision of the power animal and the strong command and invited him to use the image of the dove for healing in any way that he felt was appropriate. At this point, we used Integrative Imagery to help him create his own image of the dove. He described it to me as a beautiful grey dove with soft feathers, clear eyes and an even clearer "vision." The dove knew exactly what was needed for healing and told Jim to rest as she went inside his lungs. There, she fluttered her wings to release and dissipate all the congestion that was there.

When our session was over we discussed what had happened. Jim told me that he now felt so different from when he first entered my office that day. He described a lightness and sense of more "room" in his lungs. He said that the experience of the dove fluttering inside his lungs had such a powerful effect on him. He hesitated a moment and then said quietly, "You know, I really had the awareness of healing going on, but I also had the sense that if I were to die that the dove would just flutter out of my lungs and I would gently be transported on wings to another place."

My purpose in sharing this story is not only the power of the story itself, but also to encourage awareness that Integrative Imagery is so versatile. Even after using imagery with my clients for more than twenty-five years, I find that it continues to be a useful and awe-inspiring tool. If it can be combined with something that is as different as shamanic practice, it is possible that imagery can be combined with almost any other healing modality in such a way that it potentiates the effectiveness of both. The possibilities are limitless!

Stress Relief for Stressed-Out Nurses

By an imagery practitioner

*T*here are a multitude of simple heroes in our midst everyday; people who do their work, think outside the box, and want to make a difference. One such person is Jessica Taylor.

The amount of stress in healthcare today is so ubiquitous that this valuable use of Integrative Imagery could come from any and every hospital, nationwide. In actuality, this story took place in the surgery services of Abbott-Northwestern Medical Center in Minneapolis, MN. In a climate of increasing workload, high productivity, downsizing, and cost containment, not to mention the challenge of caring for the sick, any unit in any hospital is a scene fraught with stress.

Jessica is an evening charge nurse in peri-operative care in a surgical department that performs 90-100 surgeries a day. In the daily course of her job, Jennifer became increasingly cognizant of the mounting stress levels in herself and her co-workers. After becoming certified in Integrative Imagery, her initial desire was to introduce this modality to pre and post-operative patients. Research has consistently shown the benefits for this patient population include decreased pre and post-operative anxiety, as well as less pain and fewer narcotics to manage that pain. However, in reality there was little time or place for Jennifer to offer one-on-one imagery in this kind of clinical setting.

A more critical need seemed to be for the nurses themselves.

Jessica observed in her colleagues many tell-tale signs of stress-physical tension, headache, short temper, and anxiety, to name a few. Believing that nurses who incorporate self-care practices have less stress and provide better patient care, this nurse was compelled to do something about it. Out of necessity, combined with caring and compassion, a great idea was formed.

With management permission, Jessica scheduled three full days of individual Integrative Imagery session for nurses and support staff, totaling 27 sessions. All sessions used the technique of "transforming pain," adapted for stress. This exercise is based on the premise that with the power of the imagination, the mind can lead the body to change from one state to another, thus creating a blueprint for this change to be actualized. First, the nurses used colored pens to draw simple body diagrams of their stress. An imagery process followed which encouraged the nurse to express her state of mind/body and then transform it. In the session, each individual was given time to draw a representation of their stress level at its "worst," then a picture of "manageable stress," and then an "optimal or stress-free" state. The drawings alone often revealed very useful information as to where and how stress manifests itself. Through the relaxation and imagery process the client was then empowered to turn down the high stress level to an ideal state and then to anchor it with a "cue" in order to re-access this optimal state when needed. All participants reported positive benefits, with many continuing to use the tools on a daily basis.

In August of 2006, Jessica was nominated for and awarded hospital-wide recognition for implementing an innovative idea in her clinical setting. Recognition included being honored at a luncheon, meeting with the vice-president of the hospital, having a personal photo on the "Wall of Fame" and a $250 bonus. This champion of imagery remains determined to incorporate stress management into the work setting by proposing her job description include a set number of hours dedicated to offering stress reduction imagery sessions to her fellow staff members. A win-win for nurses and patients!

An Idea Whose Time Has Come: Hospital-Based Imagery

By imagery practitioners

*C*omplementary and Alternative Medicine (CAM) is being widely incorporated into conventional medical care throughout the country. The demand is documented by the billions of dollars the consumer spends, increasing each year. The field of CAM is so significant that the National Institute for Health has established a federal government agency to research its validity and effectiveness. The department is the National Center for Complementary and Alternative Medicine (nccam.nih.gov.) CAM encompasses dozens of practices from ancient Indian Ayurveda to Therapeutic Touch. There are four categories: mind-body medicine, biological-based practices, manipulative or body-based practices and energy-based therapies.

The mind/body modality of imagery is one of the most widely accepted therapies being incorporated into healthcare today. It is safe, effective, simple to use, accessible to everyone and cost effective. The benefits to the patient are many, including a feeling of empowerment and active participation in their own healing process. Many hospitals have made guided imagery CDs available for stress management, cancer therapy, surgery preparation and more. For example, Belleruth Naparstek's Healthjourneys CDs are being successfully used in a multitude of healthcare institutions.

Listening to a CD is a very inexpensive way to introduce guided imagery. However, it is just the beginning step. Another approach with much more impact is to incorporate trained healthcare practitioners on site to directly provide imagery services. Highlighted here are two living models illustrating integration of guided imagery specialists into a hospital-wide program.

Abbott Northwestern Hospital

Abbott Northwestern Hospital (ANW), with 650 beds, is the largest not-for-profit hospital in the Minneapolis/St Paul metropolitan area. The Institute for Health and Healing (IHH), ANW's nurse-based integrative healthcare department, provides a continuum of care for patients with inpatient, outpatient, and fitness center programs. The inpatient branch, the Integrative Medicine (IM) department, currently provides an average of 1300 patient visits per month. Practitioners are licensed and credentialed in a variety of professions including nursing, acupuncture, music therapy, massage therapy, healing touch, aromatherapy, reflexology, Reiki, and guided imagery. Five practitioners on the IHH staff are certified in Integrative Imagery.

An integral part in this comprehensive program is guided imagery. The practitioners have found that patients can access deep healing through the use of this tool by providing support and often a healthy shift in perspective for patients experiencing pain and anxiety. Imagery is offered across a full range of patient care areas throughout the hospital. Effectiveness is measured using the visual analog scale of 0-10 intensity for pain and anxiety, rated before and after an imagery session.

Referrals are received primarily from nurses and physicians. Because patients often are unfamiliar with guided imagery, there is a need for additional education and careful assessment for appropriateness and right timing when using this technique. The care provider listens for the opening when the patient talks about an imbalance such as fear, anger, anxiety, stress, sadness, grief, insomnia, and pain. Other indicators are the presence of nightmares, panic, post trauma, mention of being stuck or recurring issues. Imagery has also been shown to be useful preparing patients for surgery, for diagnostic procedures such as MRIs and scans, and for invasive medical procedures. Most commonly, patients have one or two sessions during their length of stay.

The imagery technique of finding a special place is often used as a simple introduction for patients who may feel overwhelmed by their hospital experience. Most patients can easily think of a place they would rather be than in a hospital. Occasionally someone may use the whole session just to bring a safe place into consciousness. Some have never experienced a safe place in their lives, and work hard to create one in their imaginations. The places they eventually image are unexpected and can be fun for them. This imagery provides the opportunity for them to create an accessible place within their imaginations where they can know the feeling of safety. That skill provides patients with a welcomed sense of strength, power and respite.

One example involved a severely injured farmer who was suffering embarrassment and pain during his personal care. The previous day, he had found his special place at his farm, on the deck off his kitchen, where he and his wife fed the birds. He easily slipped into the sights, sounds, smells and feel of the scene, and become quiet and peaceful. The next day as he was moaning while being bathed, he was again asked by the practitioner about the birds and he shouted, "Red! Red cardinals!" Within moments of engaging in the guided imagery, he was breathing deeply and imaging his deck, where he saw himself relaxed and calm. His bath was finished without further distress, and the nurse working with the patient even encouraged him in the session.

Integrative Imagery has also been effective in working with patients with phantom pain. A patient with a below-the-knee amputation was in anguish, and said he would try anything that might help. One technique often used is talking with an image that represents the pain. The image of pain may come in the form of a person, animal, object or even a sound or a feeling. This patient brought up an image of a navy admiral and was initially quite intimidated by the image. Eventually, he was able to work with this image of his pain and apply the insights to shift into a more peaceful relationship with his physical body. When he came out of the guided imagery, he said, "I can feel my knee. My leg ends at the knee now!"

Truly, it could be said that there is a story about guided imagery for each individual patient who uses it. The constant rediscovery of this work is that the source of all the information is within the patient. The learning accessed seems to be sitting just below the surface of consciousness, and experience shows that it is waiting to be revealed. When the patients gain clarity from the depths of their own wisdom, they know it to be their truth. That truth creates a profound opening for healing. This can also be a rewarding experience for the practitioner.

Mills-Peninsula Health Services

Dreams do sometimes come true. In the spring of 2003, Terry was asked to return to develop an imagery program at Mills-Peninsula Health Services (MPHS) in Burlingame, CA, where she had previously worked for twenty-four years. With the same name but not related to Abbott North West, the Institute for Health and Healing at MPHS offers services and education about integrative medicine, holistic health and healing practices to individuals and communities. The guided imagery clinical supervisor role quickly became a bona fide full-time, benefited position shared by two holistic nurses certified in imagery, Terry Reed and Susan Ezra.

One of the first projects was a pilot study designed to replicate the successful use of imagery in the peri-operative arena, to assess reduction of pre-operative anxiety and post-operative pain. The unique feature of the surgery preparation program is a one-hour, one-on-one session with an imagery practitioner, including the production of a customized audiotape or CD tailored to the patient's own needs and images. Although more time- consuming, this model is more powerful than just using a generic CD for the client.

The results of the study showed a significant decrease in the perception of pain and in the daily use of pain medication for the patients in the intervention group as compared to the control group.

The credibility of the outcomes laid the groundwork to offer this service to all elective surgery patients at MPHS.

Some people have no concerns regarding surgery. For most though, some degree of stress or anxiety is present. One 70 year-old woman facing a bilateral mastectomy for breast cancer was extremely anxious and distraught. Very reluctantly, she was going into the scheduled surgery that her daughter and surgeon recommended. Being "pushed into this" and feeling "scared to death" are not good attitudes under any circumstance, especially surgery. With two imagery sessions, this patient was able to cry; express her fears; find some inner strength, and create some positive, supportive images to help her accept the procedure and successfully complete the surgery.

In addition to surgery preparation, imagery services are available in MPHS's 400-bed hospital to inpatients and to outpatients to address pain, and anxiety, or to develop coping skills in dealing with acute disease or chronic conditions. Areas of care include: cancer center; critical care; chronic renal failure; chemical dependency; labor and delivery; acute rehabilitation; palliative care and medical-surgical units. Several groups and educational classes are offered to teach relaxation and guided imagery skills. Staff members are also afforded these benefits with a stress management class designed to use simple techniques for themselves and their patients at the bedside. Many of these offerings are at no-charge to in-patients as part of the "standard of excellent care" while outpatient services are on a fee for service basis or a charge for the class.

There are many other models of incorporating guided imagery into healthcare systems. Pioneering hospitals and real people are changing the face of "sick care" to true holistic health institutions. If it can happen somewhere, it can happen everywhere. We will then have the best of both worlds; active, empowered participation in our own health and well-being in the midst of expert conventional medical care. In this paradigm everyone benefits.

Section Four:
References And
Resources

The true sign of intelligence is not knowledge but imagination.
~ Albert Einstein

References

1. Watson J. Caring science as sacred science. Philadelphia: F.A. Davis Company; 2004.

2. Rossman M. Imagery: the body's natural language for healing. Alternative Therapies 2002;8 (1): 83.

3. Artress L. Walking a sacred path; rediscovering the labyrinth as a spiritual tool. New York: Riverhead Books; 1995. 111-112.

4. Heinschel JA. A descriptive study of the interactive guided imagery experience. J Holist Nurs 2002;20:325-47.

5. Heinschel JA. A descriptive study of the interactive guided imagery experience. J Holist Nurs 2002;20:337.

6. Hillhouse JE, Kiecolt-Glaser JK, & Glaser R. Stress-associated modulation of the immune response in humans. In N. Plotnifoff; 1991;Murgo r, Faith, & Wybran (eds) Stress and Immunity 3-27. Boca Raton, Fl. CRC Press.

7. Kiecolt-Glaser JF, McGuire L, Robles TF, Glaser R. Emotions and morbidity: new perspectives from psychoneuroimmunology. Annu Rev Psychol 2002; 53: 83-107.

8. Kop WJ. The integration of cardiovascular behavioral medicine and psychoneuroimmunology: new developments based on converging research fields. Brain Behav Immun 2002(4): 233-7.

9. Pert, CB. Molecules of emotion. New York: Scribner; 1997.

10. Lang E, Benolsch E, Fick L, et al. Adjunctive non-pharmacological analgesia for invasive medical procedures: a randomized trial. Lancet 2000; 355: 1486-90.

Resources

Beyond Ordinary Nursing

www.integrativeimagery.com
650-570-6157
imagine@integrativeimagery.com
Co-directors: Terry Reed, RN, MS, HN-BC and Susan Ezra, RN, HN-BC

The Certificate Program in Imagery

The Certificate Program in Imagery is a 108 contact hour training program specifically designed for licensed health care practitioners. This unique certificate program offers in-depth, hands-on training in the expanding field of Integrative Imagery, which goes beyond scripted guided imagery. It is a powerful mind/body modality that fosters active participation, returning the focus of holistic healing to the individual. The Integrative Imagery process is transformative for the practitioner and the client. Program instruction uses varied methods such as lecture, group discussion, experiential exercises and practice in pairs in small groups, with mentor guidance.

Certification

The program is endorsed by the American Holistic Nurses Association and is provider approved by the California BRN and the American Nurses Credentialing Center's Committee on Accreditation and is provider approved for Marriage & Family Therapists and Licensed Clinical Social Workers.

Program Content

Core concepts in integrative medicine, psychoneuroimmunology, and holistic healing.
Principles and theory of the Integrative Imagery process.
Stress management strategies and self-care as an integral aspect of professional practice.
Instruction in a variety of breathing and relaxation techniques.
Eight distinct Integrative Imagery techniques in Phase I - IV.

Program Benefits for Imagery Guides and Clients

Relaxation and stress management
Coping strategies
Promotion of healing
Relief of emotional/physical pain and symptoms
Control of anxiety and panic attacks
Preparation for childbirth
Preparation for surgery and medical procedures
Insights into life's purpose /career options
Accessing inner wisdom and inner resources

Course Outline

Phase I is three days and phases II through phase IV consist of an evening and three days spaced at approximately three-month intervals (Phase I through III) and six months between phases III and IV.

For details of each phase, training calendar, additional imagery benefits, special conferences, etc. see website above.

An Integrative Imagery demonstration recorded live at Phase II is available as a free MP3 download on our website.

Academy for Guided Imagery:
www.academyforguidedimagery.com
800-726-2070

Professional Associations

American Holistic Nurses Association
www.ahna.org. 800-278-2462

Imagery International
www.imageryinternational.com 707-592-7667

Listing of Certified Imagery Practitioners

www.academyforguidedimagery.com
www.imageryinternational.com
www.integrativeimagery.com

Guided Imagery CD and Audiotapes

Health Journeys: www.healthjourneys.com
Dr. Emmett Miller: www.drmiller.com
Dr. Charlotte Reznick: www.imageryforkids.com
Dr. Martin Rossman: www.thehealingmind.org
Ezra, Susan: www.integrativeimagery.com
Reed, Terry: www.integrativeimagery.com

Additional books may be ordered from
www.outskirtspress.com/guidedimageryand beyond

Bibliography

Achterberg J. Imagery in healing: shamanism and modern medicine. 2002.

Ader R. Psychoneuroimmunology: 2 vol set. MA: Elsevier; 2007.

Curran E. Guided imagery for healing children and teens. Oregon (OR); Beyond Words Publishing; 2001.

Garrison J. Imagery in you: mining for treasure in your inner world. Denver: Outskirts Press; 2006.

Heinschel JA. A descriptive study of the interactive guided imagery experience. J Holist Nurs 2002;20:325-47.

Naparstek B Invisible heroes: survivors of trauma and how they heal. New York: Bantam Dell; 2004.

Pert CB. Molecules of emotion. New York: Scribner; 1997.

Reed T. Imagery in the clinical setting: a tool for healing. Nurs Clin N Am 2007: 42: 261-277.

Rossman, ML. Fighting cancer from within. New York: Henry Holt & Co; 2003.

Rossman ML. Guided imagery for self-healing. Tiburon, CA: New World Library, 2000.

Scherwitz LW, McHenry P, Herrero R. Interactive guided imagery[SM] therapy with medical patients: predictors of health outcomes. J Altern Complement Med 2005;11(1):69-83.

Printed in the United States
115470LV00004B/154-171/P

9 781432 719746